MW01156824

Medical Readers' Theater

Medical Readers' Theater

⊙ ⊙ ⊙ ⊙ ⊙

A GUIDE

AND SCRIPTS

Edited by Todd L. Savitt

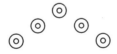

University of Iowa Press 🌱 Iowa City

University of Iowa Press, Iowa City 52242
Printed in the United States of America

http://www.uiowa.edu/~uipress

The publication of this book was generously supported by the
University of Iowa Foundation.

Printed on acid-free paper

Library of Congress Cataloging-in-Publication Data
Medical readers' theater: a guide and scripts/edited by
Todd L. Savitt.
    p.   cm.
  ISBN 0-87745-798-0 (cloth), ISBN 0-87745-799-9 (pbk.)
    1. Medicine—Drama.   2. Physicians—Drama.   3. Physician and
patient—Drama.   4. American drama—20th century.   I. Savitt,
Todd Lee, 1943– .
PS627.M42 M43   2002
812'.6080356—dc21   2002016007

02 03 04 05 06 C 5 4 3 2 1
02 03 04 05 06 P 5 4 3 2 1

*To the medical students of the Brody School of Medicine
at East Carolina University who have participated
in the Medical Readers' Theater Program:
You made it happen.*

Contents

Preface and
Acknowledgments

We have all had experiences with sickness and caregiving and physicians and medical emergencies and hospitals and doctors' offices. Our interest in matters relating to health is reflected in the many stories written on the subject. Such stories provide case examples of the kind of real-life occurrences that we can ponder and relate to our own situations. To help laypeople and medical professionals alike consider some of the issues that arise during illness, East Carolina University's Brody School of Medicine has developed a medical readers' theater program based on a number of carefully selected short stories about medicine.

Since 1988, our school has used medical readers' theater as a means both of educating health care students and professionals at the university about social and ethical issues in medicine and of establishing a dialogue about these issues with the citizens of eastern North Carolina. The concept behind our readers' theater program is simple: adapt short stories about medicine to scripts, invite medical students to serve as the readers (actors), perform the stories to public and medical audiences, and hold postperformance discussions about the issues raised by the stories with the audiences and the cast. These stories and discussions have a profound impact on both the performers and the audience members. Future physicians (cast members) have the opportunity to hear the thoughts of their future patients and their peers and teachers in the audience, and audience members have the opportunity to express their ideas and feelings about the way medicine is practiced and about crucial ethical and social issues in medicine to future physicians and to their community or professional peers.

This book provides a vehicle for those who wish to engage in discussions among citizens and professionals about important, topical issues in medicine today. The readers need not be medical students—they can be health professionals or laypeople. Anyone who can read aloud can "do" readers' theater. The only requirements are some willing readers and a good moderator for the discussions that follow the performances. Our book contains a section on how to set up a readers' theater program, followed by scripts for fourteen stories and suggested discussion questions for each story.

The ECU medical readers' theater program developed out of a grant submitted to the North Carolina Humanities Council in 1988 by Nancy King, a professor in the Department of Social Medicine at the University of North Carolina at Chapel Hill. Owing to her vision, three medical schools in North Carolina (Duke University, University of North Carolina at Chapel Hill, and East Carolina University) established medical readers' theater programs aimed at different geographical parts of the state. Initially the North Carolina Humanities Council funded the project, then administered an Exemplary Award for medical readers' theater from the National Endowment for the Humanities. When that funding expired, the dean of the medical school at East Carolina University, James A. Hallock, agreed to continue financial support of our school's medical readers' theater program.

I would like to thank Dr. Hallock for his generous support over the years. The East Carolina University Medical Foundation provided funds to purchase "ECU School of Medicine Readers' Theater Company" black T-shirts that, with blue jeans, serve as the readers' "costumes" for performances. Artistic directors Ann Bean (1988–1991) and Janice Schreiber (since 1991) patiently and expertly coached our medical student readers and, through their interpretations, imaginatively brought the scripts to life. I learned a lot from them. They opened to the students and to me a whole new realm of theater. Gregory A. Watkins of Greenville has been our primary story adapter since the beginning. All but two of the scripts in this book are the result of his creative talents. Ann Bean, mentioned above as the founding director of our ECU medical readers' theater project, adapted the other two stories. John Moskop, my colleague in the Department of Medical Humanities, has lent more than just his encouragement to the readers' theater program: he coordinated it when I was on leave and has led numerous postperformance discussions. Loretta Kopelman, chair of the Department of Medical Humanities, has supported my involvement in this medical readers' theater project from the beginning and was the first to suggest publishing the scripts. Thanks also to my colleagues in the Department of Medical Humanities, past and present, who have generously lent their time and expertise to lead discussions: Loretta Kopelman, Jeffrey Kahn, Suzanne Poirier (who also suggested several stories to adapt), Willem Landman, and Carl Elliott. Shirley Nett, my office assistant for many years, has, among other things, typed programs, compiled student bios, composed, printed, and posted countless fliers, kept track of our student readers, ordered pizzas and cokes for rehearsals, overseen arrangements at performance sites, and kept track of crucial details that would otherwise have been neglected. She does these tasks with equanimity and always with a smile. Without her the readers' theater program could not have functioned. Finally, to the students at ECU who have donated time and energy to rehearsals and performances in the midst of extremely busy and pressure-filled days, I extend a special thanks. They have been the heart and soul of this small but significant enterprise.

How to Use This Book

This book contains fourteen readers' theater scripts and groups of questions for postperformance discussions. The beauty of readers' theater is that it can be done simply. Readers do not memorize lines, move around the stage, wear costumes, or use props; their voices and facial expressions convey the meaning of the words and the story. Like radio drama, audience members imagine the scenes taking place before them.

Each script is accompanied by a cast of characters, a suggested seating arrangement for the performance, and questions for discussion. Stage directions appear in bracketed italic type. Readers will find it helpful to highlight their lines in the scripts with a light colored marker or colored pen. We suggest doing two read-throughs of a script before performing it. One person who is not a performer (e.g., the discussion leader or someone with theater or public speaking experience) should observe the rehearsal from the back of the room and make suggestions to the readers. At the actual performance, readers should, unless otherwise stated in the scripts, wear white tops and black pants or skirts (or black T-shirts and blue jeans), sit in firm but comfortable chairs with both feet on the floor, and, when they look up from their scripts, focus on a point in the back of the room (offstage focus). They should not make eye contact with the audience or turn to or look at each other, even when their characters are interacting. It is part of the audience's job to imagine what is happening. Maintaining off-stage focus takes some getting used to on the part of readers, who tend to try to sneak looks at each other or the audience while reading. Resist the temptation! Off-stage focus is *very* effective and a crucial part of readers' theater performances.

We encourage organizers of medical readers' theater programs to obtain and have participants read the original stories on which the scripts are based. This will enhance the performers' and discussion leaders' understanding of the stories. (Sources for those stories are included in the Permissions section of this book.) Our adapters have remained as true to the stories as possible, but some alterations were necessary in changing from one genre to another. In one notable case, Arthur Conan Doyle's "The Doctors of Hoyland," Gregory Watkins created two characters not in the original story to serve as narrators. The essential meaning of each story remains intact in the readers' theater script.

A further comment about remaining true to the original stories: Our adapters have retained the gender identities as they appear in the stories. We have occasionally, in our performances at ECU, experimented with switching genders of certain characters or used women to play male roles when necessity dictated (we have always had more females than males volunteer for our readers' theater program). We encourage you to experiment in similar fashion, especially as some of the stories were written at a time when female physicians were fewer in number and people's thinking about women in the medical profession differed greatly from today.

It is important to remember that the goal of doing medical readers' theater is to stimulate thinking about the issues each story raises so that audience and cast can engage in good and meaningful discussion afterward. Readers and directors should not obsess about rehearsing a story to perfection; the scripts are strong enough that the meaning and action will be clear even if readers make a mistake or two. Consider the stories as *vehicles* for the later conversations about social and ethical issues in medicine. Such an approach will also relieve some of the pressure readers might feel about performing in public. People will judge the program much less on the performance than on the power of the story and on the exchanges during the discussion.

A note about selecting sites for performances and attracting audiences: We have learned from painful experience that simply announcing (by flyer, newspaper ad, or other means of communication) the date and place of a medical readers' theater performance and discussion does *not* work. It is difficult to get people out of their homes on an evening or on a weekend afternoon or to give up a precious lunch hour to attend a program about which they know nothing. At a few of our performances, we reluctantly admit, the cast has outnumbered the audience — a real embarrassment and a waste of cast members' valuable time. Although discussions with very small audiences work quite well (everyone feels compelled to participate and lively exchanges do occur), we don't recommend the experience of playing to tiny groups. To avoid the small audience problem, it is best to arrange for performances at the regular meetings of organizations — for example, religious groups; civic, social, and book clubs; medical and other health professional societies; retirement communities; nursing homes; professional associations; community college classes; nursing and medical school classes; even lunch hours in the local hospital cafeteria. We still do a few open performances at the local bookstore or public library, primarily because we have developed a small following in the community who attend loyally.

An entire medical readers' theater program — introduction, performance, and discussion — can take as little as forty-five minutes or as long as an hour and a half. As audience members enter the room, hand each person a simple program that contains, at minimum, the title, author, and adapter of the story, the performance place and date, the sponsoring organization, and the names of (and perhaps brief biographical statements by) the readers and discussion leader. The discussion leader then begins with a welcome, a few explanatory words about readers' theater for those in the audience not familiar with the genre, and, if desired, a few biographical words (a paragraph or two at most) about the story's author. Conclude this opening segment of five to six minutes duration with a reminder that a discussion of the story among audience and cast will follow the performance and by naming the readers (usually already seated in their places). With the words, "And now, 'A Face of Stone'" (or whatever the title of the story is), the leader walks to the back of the room and the performance begins.

The actual reading lasts between ten and thirty minutes, depending on the story. When the last word of the script is read, the cast members should close their script books and the discussion leader should begin applauding to cue the audience that the reading has concluded. The leader now returns to the front of the room and stands in a prominent place that does not block the audience's view of the cast.

Here comes the trickiest part of the program — getting the audience to talk. We usually begin our discussion periods by having the discussion leader say enough words to allow the audience members a chance to compose themselves and their thoughts (especially if the story was particularly moving) and to make the transition from listeners to active participants: "I'm sure this story has stimulated your thinking about a number of matters. Now that the readers have done their job, this last part of the program depends on you. We'd like you to share your ideas and reactions to the story so all of us can gain a better understanding of it. I have a number of questions written down [wave the sheet of questions to the audience] that I can pose to you, but I'd like to start off by seeing if any of you has a comment or thought you'd like to offer. The cast will get involved in the discussion as well, but we'd like to hear from you folks a bit first. Once we've gotten into the conversation, you should feel free to pose questions to the cast about the characters they portrayed. Would anyone like to start things off?" If these inspiring words fail to bring a response from anyone in the audience, the discussion leader should ask a question — any easily answerable question about some event in the story — that will spark a member of the audience to speak up. All it takes is one person to start things off; then the rest of the group will feel relieved and begin chiming in.

Discussion leaders should not be afraid to allow several usually awkward moments of silence to elapse at the beginning. The temptation will be for the leader to fill that silence with a personal interpretation of the story. This is a mistake, for if the discussion leader falls into that trap, audience members will be much less willing to offer their own thoughts, especially if the leader is an academic scholar or physician or someone whom people might perceive as an expert on the subject under scrutiny. Also, the leader's comment might be just the opposite of what one member of the audience was about to say, thereby discouraging debate. The leader's role is to remain neutral throughout the discussion, repeating pertinent comments, asking others if they agree so as to bring out various views on an issue, calling on a variety of people so that no one dominates the discussion, turning to the cast for their comments at appropriate moments, and remaining positive and encouraging to all who raise their hands to risk expressing their thoughts in public. The goal of medical readers' theater programs is to provide a forum where citizens can consider and examine their own and others' views on issues of common concern in the medical world. People should feel comfortable sharing personal and sometimes painful experiences and debating points of contention. Discussion leaders need to keep the audience focused and deliberative but also nonconfrontational — no mean task.

We have found it best not to force the discussion in any particular direction at the beginning, but to use whatever comments the audience members start with. Once the discussion has warmed up and people begin to feel comfortable speaking, then the leader can push the audience one way or another to provoke further interactions. We have appended to each script a number of questions for the use of discussion leaders. These questions have not been placed in any particular order and can be used as the leader thinks appropriate or necessary.

When the main points of the story have received sufficient attention and/or when people seem to be getting restless, the leader should gracefully end the discussion and thank everyone for coming and participating. People ought to leave still thinking about what they have witnessed and talked about. One nice touch is to adjourn the group to a reception area where audience and cast can mingle and chat over cookies and punch to resolve concerns or discuss their thoughts further. A good ending to a fine program.

That's it. Medical readers' theater is that straightforward and easy. You can do it. Let us know how things go. We would love to hear about your experiences. Contact Todd Savitt at the Department of Medical Humanities, Brody School of Medicine at East Carolina University, Greenville, North Carolina 27858-4354; phone 252-816-2797; e-mail savittT@mail.ecu.edu.

PART I. PHYSICIANS AND PATIENTS

⊙ ⊙ ⊙ ⊙ ⊙

A Face of Stone

WILLIAM CARLOS WILLIAMS

Adapted for Readers' Theater by Gregory A. Watkins

CAST
Narrator
Doctor
Man
Woman

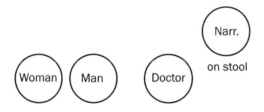

NOTES

Narrator *sits on a stool placed next to but slightly behind the doctor's chair.* Narrator *may be either male or female. Before the performance, the discussion leader should announce to the audience that the story takes place between World War I and World War II and that the narrator serves two roles: to provide continuity for the action and to express the unspoken thoughts of* Doctor.

Doctor *speaks abruptly and acts coldly toward* Man *and* Woman *until almost the very end of the story when he discovers that the woman is from Poland and suffered greatly during World War I. He then softens as he begins to put her medical condition and her concerns for her baby into the context of this history.*

Man *speaks caringly to his wife, but is frustrated by her unwillingness to communicate with the physician. He tolerates the physician's rudeness toward him and his wife and acts as a mediator between the physician and his wife.* Man *is his wife's intermediary to the outside world.*

Woman *keeps a stone face throughout the story, looking up as much as possible so the audience can see it. If she clips her words, it will sound as if she has an eastern European accent. As she says her very last line in the story, she gives a big stage smile so the audience can see the change that has taken place. This smile can be a point of discussion after the performance.*

Note to discussion leader: Physicians are as busy and harried today as they were back then when they were making house calls, seeing patients in their offices, and doing hospital rounds morning, noon, and night.

NARRATOR: As they entered his office, the doctor glanced at the clock on his wall and heaved a heavy sigh of frustration. A hurried lunch again, he thought. He motioned them to sit, and noticed that, as they did so, the man made no attempt to help his wife with her chair.

DOCTOR: What is it?

NARRATOR: He asked, looking at the child asleep in the woman's arms.

MAN: It's the baby.

NARRATOR: The doctor looked at the man. Ah, he thought, one of those fresh Jewish types, the presuming poor whose faces change the minute cash is mentioned, who take advantage of kindness at the first opportunity.

MAN: My brother told us to bring the baby to you. We already had a doctor, but he was no good.

NARRATOR: Of course.

DOCTOR: No good? How do you know he was no good? How long did you see him?

NARRATOR: Were you paying him?

DOCTOR: It doesn't matter. What did you want to see me about?

MAN: I want you to fix the baby, Doc. My brother says you're the best baby doctor around here, and this kid's sick.

DOCTOR: Well, put it on the table and take its clothes off.

NARRATOR: Neither the man nor his wife moved.

DOCTOR: *[Getting irritated]* Put the baby on the table and remove its clothes.

NARRATOR: Still, the woman wouldn't move. She sat there, staring at the doctor, holding the baby tightly to her chest. Immigrant, he thought, Italian probably. She looked dirty, like her husband, her hands and face grimy, her nails as black as her hair.

DOCTOR: *[Frustrated]* If you want me to examine the baby, you'll have to put it on the table.

MAN: *[Gently]* Gimme the baby.

NARRATOR: The woman continued to stare at the doctor, with no expression at all on her face, a face of stone. Animal distrust, the doctor thought — she's like an animal that senses danger, and is on guard against it.

MAN: *[Frustrated but still gently]* Gimme the baby.

WOMAN: *[Firmly, but without emotion]* No. I hold her.

NARRATOR: And the doctor knew, from her accent and grammar, that she had not been in this country long.

MAN: Gimme the baby. He wants to examine it.

DOCTOR: Listen. Do you want me to examine the baby or not? If you don't, I really . . .

MAN: *[Cutting Doctor off]* Wait a minute, Doc. Wait a minute.

WOMAN: You look at the throat.

DOCTOR: All right. Put the baby on the table and remove its clothing.

NARRATOR: But the woman still wouldn't move. After a moment, the doctor started twirling a pencil through the fingers of his left hand. He turned to the husband.

DOCTOR: Never mind. What's wrong with it?

MAN: She's getting thin, Doc. What do you think's the matter with her?

DOCTOR: What do you mean, "thin"?

WOMAN: Thin.

NARRATOR: The doctor turned to the woman. She flinched, but didn't move.

DOCTOR: How old is she?

WOMAN: Four months, one half.

DOCTOR: I see. And how much does she weigh?

WOMAN: Thirteen pounds, one half.

MAN: *[Translating, a bit embarrassed by his wife's speech]* Thirteen and a half pounds, Doc.

DOCTOR: That's really not that bad. How have you been feeding her?

MAN: My wife is nursing her.

WOMAN: I nurse.

DOCTOR: I see. How often do you nurse?

   [Pause, waiting for an answer]

   [Irritated] When do you nurse her?

WOMAN: When she hungry.

DOCTOR: And how often is that?

   [Pause, again waiting for an answer]

   [Irritated] How often is that?

MAN: She probably don't know, Doc.

DOCTOR: What kind of labor did she have?

MAN: I don't know. Regular, I guess.

DOCTOR: Was this her first baby?

MAN: Oh, yeah. This is her first.

NARRATOR: The doctor made a few notes on the new folder in front of him, and then stood, walked around his desk and leaned against it, facing the woman.

DOCTOR: Is the baby ever sick? Does it ever have a fever? Does it ever throw up?

WOMAN: Sometime. Sometime she throw up.

DOCTOR: How often?

   [Pause]

   [Again getting irritated when she doesn't answer] How often?

WOMAN: Sometime.

MAN: Every once in a while.

WOMAN: My milk no good?

DOCTOR: Not necessarily. Let me see the baby.

NARRATOR: The doctor leaned forward, reaching for the baby. It took one look at him and let out a wild scream. The woman clutched the child to her breast, stood, and turned for the door.

WOMAN: Baby scared. We go now.

DOCTOR: Oh, Christ.

MAN: *[Frustrated, but caringly]* Don't be so scared. He ain't gonna hurt you. *[To Doctor]* I'm sorry, Doc, but she ain't been in this country long and she's afraid you're gonna hurt the baby.

NARRATOR: The man turned and went to his wife.

MAN: *[Gently coaxing her]* Gimme the baby.

NARRATOR: He took the child from her arms and carried it to the table, removed its clothing, and stepped back to give the doctor room to examine it.

MAN: You look at the baby, Doc. I'll keep the wife out of your way.

NARRATOR: The doctor looked at the still-screaming infant and could find nothing wrong with it, other than the natural results of foolish, irregular routine, and, probably, insufficient breast milk. He handed the child and its clothing to its mother, who huddled by the door and dressed it.

DOCTOR: There's nothing wrong with the baby. But she does need to be fed on a regular schedule. You explain that to your wife.

MAN: You got it, Doc.

DOCTOR: And the baby will need some formula to supplement the mother's milk. Get some, and see to it that the baby gets it on a regular schedule.

MAN: Okay, Doc.

WOMAN: We go?

MAN: Yeah, we go. Thanks, Doc. You're a good guy.

NARRATOR: The man reached into his pocket and pulled out a small wad of crumpled bills.

MAN: How much we owe you, Doc?

DOCTOR: Three dollars.

MAN: Oy, Doc. I'm a working man. I can't afford . . .

WOMAN: *[Cutting him off]* Please we go.

MAN: Okay, okay. Look, Doc, I want to be fair, 'cause you done right by us for sure, but I really can't handle more than a couple of bucks.

DOCTOR: That'll be fine. Now, I really am very busy . . .

MAN: Sure, sure, Doc. Here you go.

NARRATOR: The man laid the money neatly on the doctor's desk, turned, and joined his wife at the door.

MAN: By the way, Doc. If we need you anytime I want you to come out to the house and see it. You gotta watch this kid.

NARRATOR: Ah, the doctor thought, but of course.

DOCTOR: I don't know. Where do you live?

MAN: 1317 Marsh. Out in West End. Near the old warehouse district.

NARRATOR: Near the dumps, the doctor thought.

DOCTOR: I'll come out if you give me decent warning. Call me in the morning. And don't call me out there every time the kid gets a bellyache. Or because your wife thinks it's dying. Or at dinnertime, or at two in the morning, or in the middle of a snowstorm. I'm telling you now so you'll know. I've got more than enough to do already.

MAN: Okay, Doc. But you come.

DOCTOR: Only under those conditions.

WOMAN: We go now.

MAN: Yeah, yeah. It's a deal, Doc. Bye now.

DOCTOR: Goodbye.

NARRATOR: And the man and his wife, and their child, turned and left. [Pause] And sure enough, on a Sunday night, at nine o'clock, with the thermometer at six below and the roads like long, black skating rinks, they called the doctor at his home.

DOCTOR: Nothing doing.

MAN: But Doc, you said you'd come.

DOCTOR: I'm not coming out there tonight. I won't do it. I'll ask my associate to make the call, or maybe some good, younger man who lives in the neighborhood. But I'm not coming over there tonight.

MAN: But we need you, Doc. The baby's very sick.

DOCTOR: I can't help it. I'm not coming.

NARRATOR: "Who in the world are you talking to like that?" his wife asked. "You mustn't do that."

DOCTOR: Leave me alone. I know what I'm doing.

NARRATOR: "But my dear," she said.

DOCTOR: *[Irritated]* I *know* what I'm doing.

   [Pause]

NARRATOR: Four months passed. On the first warm day in April, about twenty women came to the doctor's office, all with babies. He started at 1 P.M., and by three o'clock was still going strong.

DOCTOR: Anybody left out there?

NARRATOR: he asked the woman he thought was his last patient. "Oh yes," she said, "there's a couple out there with a baby."

DOCTOR: Oh, Lord. It's half past three and I still have house calls to make.

MAN: Hello, Doc.

NARRATOR: And there they were. The same fresh, Jewish grin. The same face of stone, still holding the baby. But the child had grown to twice its former size. At first, the doctor didn't remember them, but only for a moment.

DOCTOR: *[Coldly—he's not happy to see them]* Oh, hello. What can I do for you?

NARRATOR: And make it snappy.

MAN: We just want you to look at the baby, Doc.

DOCTOR: Oh.

MAN: *[Picking up on Doctor's unwelcoming attitude, but trying not to sound annoyed himself]* Listen, Doc. We've been waiting out there two hours.

NARRATOR: Oh, for Christ's . . .

DOCTOR: *[Still irritated, impatient]* All right. Put it on the table. Come on.

NARRATOR: And as the man did so, the doctor noticed a cluster of red pimples near the man's right eyebrow, reaching to the bridge of his nose. Like bedbug bites, he thought. No doubt he'll want me to do something about them before they leave.

DOCTOR: Well? What's the matter, now?

MAN: It's the baby, Doc.

DOCTOR: I had assumed as much. Well? What's the matter with it? It looks perfectly fine to me.

NARRATOR: And it did. About ten months old, with a round, happy face.

MAN: Yeah, but her body isn't so good.

WOMAN: You examine all over.

NARRATOR: Of course.

DOCTOR: Do you realize what time it is?

MAN: Shouldn't we take her clothes off?

DOCTOR: I suppose.

NARRATOR: So the wife began to remove the baby's clothing, and the doctor sat down and started taking notes.

DOCTOR: How old is it?

MAN: *[Repeating question to his wife]* How old is it?

WOMAN: Ten month. Next Tuesday ten month.

NARRATOR: Her expression, no expression, never changing.

DOCTOR: Are you still nursing it?

WOMAN: Sure. She won't take bottle.

DOCTOR: *[Getting agitated]* Do you mean to say that after what I told you last time you still haven't weaned the baby?

MAN: What can we do, Doc? We tried, but she just won't let go of the breast. You can't make her take the bottle.

DOCTOR: Does she eat?

MAN: Yeah. A little. But she won't take much.

DOCTOR: Cod liver oil?

MAN: She takes it all right, but she spits it back up half an hour later. We stopped giving it to her.

DOCTOR: Orange juice?

MAN: Oh, sure. Most of the time.

DOCTOR: So she's been nursing and eating a little cereal. And that's all.

MAN: Uh, yeah, that's about it.

DOCTOR: And how often does she nurse?

MAN: Whenever she wants to. Sometimes every two hours. Sometimes she just sleeps. Like that.

DOCTOR: Didn't I tell you to feed her regularly?

MAN: We can't do that, Doc. The baby cries, my wife gives it to her.

NARRATOR: *[Calming himself]* Patience.

DOCTOR: Why don't you put it in a crib?

MAN: My wife won't give it up. That's the way she is, Doc. What can I say? She won't do no different. She wants the baby next to her so she can feel it.

NARRATOR: The doctor turned to the woman, still standing at the table.

DOCTOR: Have you got it undressed?

WOMAN: You want shoe off?

NARRATOR: He stood, and went to the table.

DOCTOR: Excuse me.

NARRATOR: He pulled the child's shoes and socks off together. He picked the baby up, by the ankles and back of the neck, and carried it to the scales. The woman followed him closely, watching his every move. The baby, apparently much calmer than her mother, merely sagged, smiling in his grasp. He looked down at her clean, happy face and returned her smile, amused in spite of himself.

DOCTOR: Twenty pounds, four ounces. What do you want for a ten-month-old? There's nothing wrong with her. Put her clothes back on.

WOMAN: You examine her first.

NARRATOR: The doctor's face reddened slightly, but the woman ignored him.

WOMAN: She too thin. Look her body.

DOCTOR: Very well.

NARRATOR: The doctor returned the child to the table, fetched his stethoscope, and went rapidly over her chest.

DOCTOR: *[Impatient]* She's fine. No rickets. No problems. Now, please get her dressed. I have a lot to do yet this afternoon.

NARRATOR: The woman hesitated.

WOMAN: She all right?

NARRATOR: She asked. Only with her voice. Her face remained completely expressionless, her eyes a brittle, pale green. The doctor found himself searching his memory for another like it. One he had seen in a painting, perhaps — Mantegna, or Botticelli. He shook his head.

DOCTOR: Yes. But for God's sake get her off the breast. Feed her exactly the way I told you to.

WOMAN: No will take bottle.

DOCTOR: Fine. I don't give a damn about the bottle. Feed her from a cup, from a spoon, any way at all. But feed her regularly. That's all.

NARRATOR: The doctor turned and went to the sink. While he washed his hands, the woman dressed her baby, clutched it to her chest, and walked to the door. Her husband hovered near the sink, and caught the doctor as he turned to go to his desk.

DOCTOR: What?

MAN: *[In a stage whisper]* Doc,

NARRATOR: he said, too quietly for his wife to hear.

MAN: I want you to examine my wife.

DOCTOR: What the — what the hell do you think I am? Don't you know . . .

MAN: *[Cutting him off]* We waited two hours and ten minutes for you, Doc. Just look her over and see what the matter with her is.

NARRATOR: The unmitigated audacity, he thought. But he turned and looked at the woman, still standing at his office door, her baby in her arms. What a creature, he thought, what a face, and what a body. He considered the tear in her dress, a triangular rip above the left knee.

DOCTOR: Sit. *[Pause]* Sit.

NARRATOR: He gestured for both of them to take seats. The husband did so immediately, the wife after a long, curious look at both men. What the hell, the doctor thought, no use getting excited with people like these. With anyone, for that matter. All you can do is what you can do. He took his seat at the desk.

DOCTOR: Go ahead. What's the matter with her?

MAN: She gets pains in her legs. Especially at night. And she's got a spot near her right knee. It came last week, a big blue-looking thing.

DOCTOR: Has she ever had rheumatism?

NARRATOR: The man shrugged.

DOCTOR: You know, go to bed with swollen joints? Lasts about six weeks?

NARRATOR: Both men looked to the wife.

DOCTOR: Have you had rheumatism?

[Pause]

MAN: *[Embarrassed]* She don't know.

NARRATOR: The man's face colored slightly. The doctor had noticed it before, but could not remember the exact circumstances. He turned again to the wife.

DOCTOR: Tell her to open her dress.

MAN: *[Gently]* Open your dress.

NARRATOR: She did so, slowly and reluctantly, after handing the baby to her husband. She turned and faced the doctor, who came around his desk to where she stood.

DOCTOR: Let me see your legs. The left one first.

NARRATOR: She untied the white rags just above her knees and let her black stockings fall to her ankles. Her legs were oddly bowed, like Turkish scimitars, flattened and somewhat rotated on themselves.

DOCTOR: You had rickets, late in your childhood.

NARRATOR: She didn't answer — just stood there. Her legs, while they did not look weak, were as ugly and misshapen as useful legs could be in a woman so young. The doctor noticed a large discolored area near her left knee.

DOCTOR: That spot comes from a broken varicose vein.

MAN: Yeah, I thought so. She's got them all up both legs.

DOCTOR: That's from carrying a child.

MAN: Oh, no. She had them before that. They been that way since I've known her. Is that what makes her legs hurt?

DOCTOR: I don't think so.

NARRATOR: The doctor took each of the woman's legs in his hands, and looked at them carefully.

DOCTOR: No, I don't think so.

MAN: What is it, then? It hurts her real bad, especially at night.

DOCTOR: Well, in the first place, she's bowlegged as hell. That throws the strain where it doesn't belong. And look at those shoes.

MAN: Yeah, I know.

NARRATOR: She was wearing a pair of fancy high-heeled slippers — evening wear. They were worn, and badly broken down.

DOCTOR: I don't see how she can walk in them.

MAN: That's what I told her. I wanted her to get a pair of shoes that fit, but she wouldn't do it.

DOCTOR: Well, she's got to do it.

NARRATOR: He turned to her.

DOCTOR: Throw away these shoes. Get shoes with flat heels — Cuban heels if you must. But new shoes. *[To Man]* How old is she?

NARRATOR: Her husband again reddened slightly.

MAN: Twenty-four.

DOCTOR: Where was she born?

MAN: In Poland.

DOCTOR: *[Surprised]* Poland? Are you sure?

MAN: Yeah. Why?

DOCTOR: *[Takes this slowly. Realization dawns as he works this out in his mind and she becomes a person to him.]*
Well. Twenty-four years old, you say. That's different. That's probably the explanation for her legs. She must have been a little girl during the war, maybe five or six years old.

NARRATOR: He turned to the woman.

DOCTOR: Is that right?

NARRATOR: She didn't answer. Or wouldn't. Or couldn't.

DOCTOR: What did you get to eat?

NARRATOR: If she heard him, she gave no sign. She turned to her husband.

DOCTOR: Did she lose anyone during the war?

MAN: Everyone. She lost everybody.

DOCTOR: How did she get over here, then?

MAN: She came over four years ago. She has a sister here.

NARRATOR: So that's it, the doctor thought, watching her take her baby from her husband's arms, watching her fussing with it, cooing at it, paying no attention whatsoever to anyone else in the room. No wonder she's built the way she is. What she went through over there . . .

MAN: What are we gonna do about her pain, Doc?

DOCTOR: Get her some decent shoes. Do that right away.

MAN: Okay, Doc.

DOCTOR: *[Softening]* She could be operated on, for those veins, but I wouldn't advise it. Not yet, anyway. Get one of those woven elastic bandages, a three-inch one. They're inexpensive and they'll help.

MAN: Doc, can't you give her some pills to stop the pain?

DOCTOR: *[Hastily]* No, not me. But I think you should get her teeth looked at, maybe. If you want to. That kind of thing. And *[Reconsidering]* — damn. Okay. I'll give you something. It's not dope, you understand? It will only help if there's some rheumatism connected with her pain.

NARRATOR: The doctor turned to the woman, and waved to get her attention.

DOCTOR: Can you swallow a pill?

WOMAN: How big?

MAN: She swallows an aspirin when I give it to her, but she usually puts it in a spoonful of water first, to dissolve it.

NARRATOR: Once again the little man reddened, and the doctor saw, for the first time, the nature of the love he felt for his wife, and the extent of her reliance on him.

DOCTOR: *[Gently]* They're pretty big pills. Look, they're green. That's a coating that keeps them from upsetting your stomach.

WOMAN: Let me see.

NARRATOR: She held out her hand to the doctor, and he placed a few of the pills in her palm.

WOMAN: For pains in leg?

DOCTOR: Yes.

NARRATOR: She looked at the pills in her hand for a moment, then back at the doctor. And for the first time since she had entered his office, several months past, she smiled.

WOMAN: *[Big stage smile]* Yes. I take them.

END

QUESTIONS FOR DISCUSSION

Is this any way to treat a patient? Was the physician justified in acting the way he did toward the couple?

Were the couple good patients?

Why did the physician dislike this couple? Is it appropriate and/or acceptable for physicians to dislike (or have other feelings about) patients?

Who was the patient during each visit? Who do you think instigated each of the visits? Cite evidence for your view. Why did the couple come to the doctor each time? Cite evidence.

Why did the physician change his demeanor toward the patients near the end of the story? At what specific point do you think he changed? Did he change for good — that is, did he learn a lesson — or do you think he just changed for this couple alone?

Why did the woman act the way she did toward the baby? Was the baby sick?

What was the role of the man in the story? What was the nature of the relationship between the man and the woman? Why did the man tolerate the physician's rudeness with such equanimity?

Why did the woman finally smile?

To whom does the title of the story refer?

This story takes place between World War I and World War II. Is it dated or does it still ring true today? What message do you take away from the story?

Do you think race, ethnicity, gender, sexual orientation, or socioeconomic status play a role in the way physicians, nurses, and other health care professionals deal with patients today?

This physician stereotyped the couple as soon as they walked in the door. Were his assumptions about the couple based on these stereotypes correct? Is stereotyping ever useful for health professionals or for others in various situations?

The Girl with a Pimply Face

WILLIAM CARLOS WILLIAMS

Adapted for Readers' Theater by Gregory A. Watkins

CAST
Narrator
Doctor
Young Girl
Mother
Woman
Doctor's Wife
Father
Second Doctor

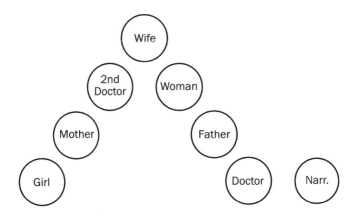

NOTES

If desired Father *and* Second Doctor *can be played by one reader, and* Doctor's Wife *and* Woman *by one reader. The person reading the part of* Young Girl

should chew gum throughout the performance. Before the performance, the dis-
cussion leader should announce to the audience that the Narrator *serves two*
roles: to provide continuity for the action and to express the unspoken thoughts of
Doctor.

NARRATOR: A local druggist sent in the call: 50 Summer Street, second
    floor, the door to the left. A baby just brought home from the hospi-
    tal. Apparently in pretty bad condition. It was half past twelve and I
    had just sat down to lunch.
DOCTOR: Can't they wait 'til after office hours?
NARRATOR: I asked. But no. They're foreigners and you know how they
    are. All the same. "Please come now!"
DOCTOR: Ah, well. The baby must be pretty bad.
NARRATOR: It was two-thirty when I got to the place, over a shop in the
    business part of town. One of those street doors between plate-glass
    show windows. A narrow entry with smashed mail boxes on one side
    and a dark stair leading straight up. I'd been to the address a number of
    times during the past few years to see various people who had lived
    there.
DOCTOR: *[Stands]* Hmm. No doorbell.
NARRATOR: I knocked vigorously on the wavy-glass door panel to the left.
    The kitchen door, as I remembered, was at the rear of the apartment.
YOUNG GIRL: *[Stands, always chewing gum, with feet apart, head cocked, face
    and voice expressionless (like she has "an attitude")]* Come in.
NARRATOR: I opened the door and saw a lank-haired girl of about fifteen,
    standing beside the table, chewing gum and eyeing me curiously. Her
    hair was coal-black, and one of her eyelids drooped a little.
YOUNG GIRL: Well? What do you want?
NARRATOR: There was a hard, straight thing about her that gave an im-
    pression of excellence. A tough, no-kidding quality.
DOCTOR: I'm the doctor.
YOUNG GIRL: Oh, you're the doctor. The baby's inside. *[Pause]* Want to
    see her?

DOCTOR: *[Surprised at her question]* Sure. That's what I'm here for. *[Pause — puzzled, trying to figure out what's going on here]* Where's your mother?

YOUNG GIRL: Out. I don't know when she's coming back. But you can take a look at the baby if you want to.

DOCTOR: Let's see her.

NARRATOR: She led the way into the bedroom, toward the front of the flat. The room was unlit, the only windows being those in the kitchen and along the facade of the building.

YOUNG GIRL: There she is.

NARRATOR: I looked on the bed and saw a small face, emaciated and quiet — unnaturally quiet — sticking out of the open end of a tightly rolled blue cotton blanket. The whole bundle — blanket and child — wasn't much larger than a good-sized loaf of bread. Only the baby's yellowish face showed, tightly hatted and framed by a corner of the blanket.

DOCTOR: What's the matter with her?

YOUNG GIRL: *[Indifferent throughout this scene]* I dunno.

NARRATOR: I looked again at the girl. She was fresh as paint and seemed as indifferent to her sister as if the child were no relation at all. My amusement must have been apparent. She looked back at me, chewing her gum vigorously, standing with her feet well apart. She cocked her head and looked me straight in the eye.

YOUNG GIRL: Well?

NARRATOR: She had one of those small, squeezed-up faces — snub nose, overhanging eyebrows, and a terrible complexion, pimply and coarse.

DOCTOR: When's your mother coming back, do you think?

YOUNG GIRL: Maybe in an hour. But maybe you better come when my father's here. He talks English. *[Pause]* He ought to come in around five, I guess.

DOCTOR: Can't you tell me something about the baby? *[Pause, waiting for Girl to answer. This whole encounter with the Girl is awkward.]* I hear it's been sick. *[Pause, waiting for Girl to answer]* Does it have a fever?

YOUNG GIRL: I dunno.

DOCTOR: Does it have diarrhea? *[Long pause]* Are its movements green?

YOUNG GIRL: Sure, I guess so. It was in the hospital, but it got worse so my father brought it home today.

NARRATOR: There was a cold bottle of half-finished milk lying on the coverlet, the nipple-end hidden behind the baby's head.

DOCTOR: How old is she? *[Pause. Tries again.]* It's a girl, did you say?

YOUNG GIRL: Yeah, it's a girl.

DOCTOR: Your sister?

YOUNG GIRL: Sure. *[Pause]* You want to examine it?

DOCTOR: No, thanks.

NARRATOR: For the moment I had lost all interest in the baby. This young kid in charge of the house did something to me that I liked. She was just a child, but nobody was putting anything over on her if she knew it. But the *real* thing about her was the complete lack of the smell of a liar. She wasn't in the least presumptive. Just straight.

YOUNG GIRL: Okay.

NARRATOR: Of course, she wasn't such a child. She had breasts I knew would be like small stones to the hand, good muscular arms and fine hard legs. Her bare feet were stuck into broken-down leather sandals, like the ones you see on children at the beach in summer. She was heavily tanned, too, wherever her skin showed. Just one of the kids you'd find loafing around the pools they have outside towns and cities everywhere these days. A tough little nut finding her own way in the world.

DOCTOR: What's the matter with your legs?

NARRATOR: They were bare, and covered with scabby sores.

YOUNG GIRL: Poison ivy. You ought to have seen it two days ago. This ain't nothing. *[Pause]* You're a doctor. What can I do for it?

DOCTOR: Let's see it.

NARRATOR: She put her leg up on a chair and pulled back her skirt. *[Girl sits.]* She had been badly bitten by mosquitoes, as I saw it, but she insisted on poison ivy. She had scratched at the affected places with her nails, and that's what made it look worse.

DOCTOR: That's not so bad. You should leave it alone, stop scratching it.

YOUNG GIRL: Yeah, I know that, but I can't. Scratching's the only thing makes it feel better.

DOCTOR: What's that on your foot?

YOUNG GIRL: What?

DOCTOR: That big, brown spot on the back of your foot.

YOUNG GIRL: Dirt, I guess.

DOCTOR: Why don't you wash it?

YOUNG GIRL: I do.

NARRATOR: Her gum chewing never stopped, and her fixed nonexpression never changed.

YOUNG GIRL: Say, what could I do for my face?

NARRATOR: I looked at her closely.

DOCTOR: *[Sits]* You have what they call acne. All those blackheads and pimples you see there. *[Pause]* Let's see. The first thing you ought to do, I suppose, is to get some good soap.

YOUNG GIRL: What kind of soap? Lifebuoy?

DOCTOR: No, no. I'd suggest one of those cakes of Lux. Not the flakes but the cake.

YOUNG GIRL: Yeah, I know. Three for seventeen.

DOCTOR: Use it every morning. Bathe your face in very hot water. You know, until the skin is red from it. That's to bring the blood up to the surface. Then take a piece of ice . . . you have ice, don't you?

YOUNG GIRL: Sure.

DOCTOR: Hold it in a face cloth, or whatever you have, and rub that all over your face. Do that right after you've washed it in the very hot water, before it has cooled. Rub the ice all over. Do that every day for a month and your skin will improve. *[Pause]* If you like, you can use some cold cream once in a while. Not much, just a little, and rub that in last of all, if your face feels too dry.

YOUNG GIRL: Will that help me?

DOCTOR: If you stick to it, it'll help you.

YOUNG GIRL: All right.

DOCTOR: There's a lotion I could give you to use along with that. Remind me of it when I come back later. *[Pause]* Why aren't you in school?

YOUNG GIRL: I'm not going anymore. They can't make me. Can they?

DOCTOR: They can try.

YOUNG GIRL: How can they? I know a girl thirteen that don't go and they can't make her either.

DOCTOR: Don't you want to learn things?

YOUNG GIRL: I know enough already.

DOCTOR: Are you going to get a job?

YOUNG GIRL: I got a job here. Looking after the Jews across the hall. They give me three-fifty a week, all summer.

DOCTOR: Good for you. *[Pause]* You think your father'll be here around five? *[Stands]*

YOUNG GIRL: Guess so. He ought to be.

DOCTOR: I'll come back then.

YOUNG GIRL: All right.

[Doctor turns upstage.]

NARRATOR: I came back at five-thirty, once more climbed the wooden stairs, and knocked on the kitchen door.

[Doctor turns downstage. Girl, Mother, and Woman stand.]

MOTHER: *[With a Russian accent]* Come in.

NARRATOR: I opened the door and entered. An impressive, bulky woman, growing toward fifty, in a black dress, with graying hair and a long, seamed face stood by the table. The mother. Beside her stood a younger, plumpish woman with blond hair, well cared for, in a neat house-dress — as if she had dolled herself up just for the occasion. The girl I had met earlier stood behind the older women. No one spoke.

DOCTOR: Hello.

NARRATOR: I aimed the greeting at the young girl, but she didn't answer.

MOTHER: *[Always with a Russian accent. She is melodramatic (almost hysterical) through entire scene.]* Doctor, save my baby. She very sick.

NARRATOR: The woman spoke with a thick, heavy voice, and seemed overcome with grief.

MOTHER: Doctor. Doctor.

DOCTOR: All right, all right, let's take a look at her.

[All sit.]

NARRATOR: Everybody headed toward the front of the house, the mother in the lead. I lagged behind to speak to the second woman, the interpreter.

DOCTOR: What happened?

WOMAN: The baby was not doing well so they took it to the hospital, to see if the doctors there could help it. It got worse. Her husband took it out this morning. It looks bad to me.

MOTHER: Yes. Me got seven children. One daughter married. This my baby.

NARRATOR: She pointed at the child on the bed, and wiped her face with the back of her hand.

MOTHER: [Becomes frantic during this speech] This baby no do good. Me almost crazy. Don't know who can help. What doctor, I don't know. Somebody tell me take to hospital. I think maybe do some good. Five days she there. Cost me two dollar every day, ten dollar. I got no money. When I see my baby, she worse. She look dead. I no can leave she there. No. No. I say everybody, no. I take she home. Doctor, you save my baby. I pay you, I pay you everything.

DOCTOR: Wait a minute, wait a minute.

NARRATOR: I turned to the other woman.

DOCTOR: What happened?

WOMAN: The baby got diarrhea in the hospital. And she was all dirty when they went to see her. They got all excited.

MOTHER: All sore behind . . .

NARRATOR: The young woman said a few words to her in a language that sounded like Russian, but it didn't stop her.

MOTHER: [Frantic] No, no. I send she to hospital, and when I see she like that I can't leave she there. My babies no that way. Never. I take she home.

DOCTOR: Take your time, take your time. [Pause] Take off her clothes. Everything off. [Pause] This is a regular party. It's certainly warm enough in here. Does she vomit?

MOTHER: She no eat. How can she vomit?

WOMAN: Yes. The nurse said she was vomiting in the hospital.

NARRATOR: We had been having a lot of such cases in my hospital, an infectious diarrhea that practically all the children got when they came in for any cause. I supposed that that was what had happened to the child. No doubt it had been in a bad way before that, what with improper feeding and all, and when they took it in the diarrhea had developed. Sometimes these things don't turn out so well.

DOCTOR: You're lucky you brought it home when you did. One nurse for ten or twenty babies. They do all they can but you can't run and change the whole ward every five minutes.

NARRATOR: The infant looked too lifeless, though, for diarrhea to be the only problem.

MOTHER: You want all clothes off?

DOCTOR: Everything off.

NARRATOR: And there it lay, just skin and bones with a round, fleshless head, and the usual potbelly you find in such cases. The mother turned it over so I could see its reddened buttocks.

MOTHER: Look. What kind of nurse that? My babies never that way.

DOCTOR: Take your time. It's really not that bad.

NARRATOR: And it wasn't. Any child with loose movements might have had the same half an hour after being cared for.

DOCTOR: Come on, move away. Give me a chance. You keep hovering over the baby as if you're afraid I might expose it.

NARRATOR: It had no temperature. There was no rash. The mouth was in reasonably good shape. Eyes, ears negative. The moment I put my stethoscope to the little bony chest, however, the whole thing became clear. The infant had a severe congenital heart defect, a roar when you listened over the heart that meant, to put it crudely, that she was no good, never would be. I looked at the mother.

DOCTOR: She's got a bad heart.

NARRATOR: She began to blubber.

DOCTOR: I'll help her. But she's got a bad heart. That will never be any better.

MOTHER: I give you anything. I pay you. I pay you twenty dollar. Doctor, you fix my baby. You good doctor. You fix.

DOCTOR: All right, all right. [Pause] What are you feeding it?

NARRATOR: They told me, and it was a ridiculous formula, unboiled besides. I regulated it properly for them, and told them how to make it up. I looked to the young girl.

DOCTOR: Have you got enough bottles?

YOUNG GIRL: Sure, we got bottles.

DOCTOR: Okay. Then go ahead.

MOTHER: You think you cure she?

NARRATOR: The mother was at me again, crying, so different from her tough female fifteen-year-old.

DOCTOR: [Stands] You do what I tell you for three days, and I'll come back and see how you're getting on.

MOTHER: [Stands] Thank you doctor. So much. I pay you. I got today no money. I pay ten dollar to hospital. They cheat me. I got no more money. I pay you Friday when my husband get pay. You save my baby.

NARRATOR: What a woman! I couldn't get away.

MOTHER: She my baby, doctor. I no want to lose. Me got seven children. . .

DOCTOR: Yes, you told me.

MOTHER: But this my baby. You understand? She very sick. You good doctor.

NARRATOR: To get away from her I turned again to the young girl.

DOCTOR: You better get going after more bottles, before the stores close. I'll come back Friday morning.

YOUNG GIRL: How about that stuff for my face you were gonna give me?

DOCTOR: That's right. Wait a minute.

NARRATOR: I sat down on the edge of the bed to write out a prescription for an acne lotion. The two older women looked at me in surprise — wondering, I suppose, how I knew the girl. I finished writing the prescription and handed it to her.

DOCTOR: Sop it on your face at bedtime and let it dry on. Don't get it in your eyes.

YOUNG GIRL: I won't.

DOCTOR: I'll see you in a couple of days.

MOTHER: Doctor, you come back. I pay you. But all a time short. Always tomorrow come milk man. Must pay rent, must pay coal, got no money.

Too much cook, too much wash, too much work. Nobody help. I don't know what's a matter. This door, doctor, this door. This house make sick. Make sick.

DOCTOR: I'll do the best I can.

[Mother sits.]

NARRATOR: And I left. The young girl followed me onto the stairs.

[Girl stands.]

YOUNG GIRL: How much is this gonna cost?

NARRATOR: She looked at me shrewdly, the prescription in her hand.

DOCTOR: Not much. Tell them you only got half a dollar. Tell them I said that's all it's worth.

YOUNG GIRL: Is that right?

DOCTOR: Absolutely. Don't pay a cent more for it.

YOUNG GIRL: Say, you're all right.

NARRATOR: She looked at me appreciatively.

DOCTOR: Have you got half a dollar?

YOUNG GIRL: Sure, why not?

[Girl sits.]

NARRATOR: That evening, my wife asked me about the case. *[Wife stands.]* She had heard about it.

DOCTOR: I met a wonderful girl.

DOCTOR'S WIFE: What? Another?

DOCTOR: Some tough baby. I'm crazy about her. Talk about straight stuff.

NARRATOR: I described the case to her, and told her what I'd done.

DOCTOR: The mother's an odd one, too. I don't quite make her out.

DOCTOR'S WIFE: Did they pay you?

DOCTOR: No. I don't suppose they have any cash.

DOCTOR'S WIFE: Well, I don't see why you have to do all this charity work. This is a case you should report to the Emergency Relief. You'll get at least two dollars a call from them.

DOCTOR: The father has a job, I understand. That counts me out.

DOCTOR'S WIFE: What sort of job?

DOCTOR: I dunno. Forgot to ask.

DOCTOR'S WIFE: What's the baby's name? So I can put it in the book.

DOCTOR: Damn. I never thought to ask them that, either. I think they must have told me but I can't remember it. Some kind of a Russian name.

DOCTOR'S WIFE: You are the limit. Honestly! Who are they anyhow?

DOCTOR: You know, I think it must be the family Kate was telling us about. You remember? The time the little kid was playing one afternoon after school, and fell down the front steps and knocked herself unconscious.

DOCTOR'S WIFE: I don't recall.

DOCTOR: Sure you do. That's the family. I get it now. Kate took the brat down there in a taxi and went up with her to see that everything was all right. Yeah, that's it. The old woman took the older child by the hair, because she hadn't watched her sister, and gave her a hell of a beating. Don't you remember Kate telling us afterward? She thought the old woman was going to murder the child, she screamed and threw her around so. Some old gal. You can see they're all afraid of her. What a world! I suppose the damned brat drives her cuckoo. But boy, how she clings to that baby.

DOCTOR'S WIFE: The last hope, I suppose.

DOCTOR: Yeah, and the worst bet in the lot. There's a break for you.

DOCTOR'S WIFE: She'll love it, just the same.

DOCTOR: More, usually.

[Wife sits.]

NARRATOR: Three days later I called at the flat again.

[Father stands.]

FATHER: Come in.

NARRATOR: I entered. By the kitchen table stood a short, thickset man in baggy working pants and a heavy cotton undershirt. He seemed to have the stability of a cube placed on one of its facets—a smooth, highly colored Slavic face, long black moustaches widely separated, and perfectly candid blue eyes. By his look he reminded me at once of his daughter, absolutely unruffled. The shoulders of an ox.

FATHER: You the doctor? Come in.

NARRATOR: The young girl was beside him, the mother in the bedroom.

DOCTOR: How's the baby?

FATHER: No better. Won't eat.

DOCTOR: How are its bowels?

FATHER: Not so bad.

DOCTOR: Does it vomit?

FATHER: No.

DOCTOR: Then it *is* better.

NARRATOR: By this time the mother had heard us and come into the room. She seemed worse than the last time. Absolutely inconsolable.

[Mother stands.]

MOTHER: Doctor, doctor.

NARRATOR: I put her aside and went in to the baby.

DOCTOR: It's better. Much better.

NARRATOR: The heart, of course, was the same.

MOTHER: How she heart? Today little better?

NARRATOR: I started to explain things to the father, but as soon as his wife got the drift of what I was saying she was all over me again. The tears began to pour. There was no use talking.

MOTHER: Doctor, you good doctor. You do something fix my baby.

NARRATOR: She took my left hand in both of hers and kissed it through her tears. As she did so I finally realized she'd been drinking. I turned to the man, who stood red-faced, watching his wife indifferently, then back to the woman. I began to feel deeply sorry for her.

[Mother and Father sit.]

DOCTOR: *[To himself]* Hell! Damn it! The sons of bitches. Why do these things have to be? *[Doctor turns upstage.]*

NARRATOR: The next day I came into the coatroom at the hospital where several of the visiting staff were standing around smoking. They were talking about a hunting dog that belonged to one of the doctors. It had come down with distemper and seemed likely to die.

[Second Doctor stands; Doctor turns downstage.]

SECOND DOCTOR: I called up half a dozen vets around here, and do you know how much they wanted to charge me for giving the serum to that animal? They had the nerve to charge me five dollars a shot for it! Can you beat that? Five dollars a shot!

DOCTOR: Did you give them the job?

SECOND DOCTOR: I should say not! But can you beat that? We're nothing but a bunch of slop-heels compared to those guys. We deserve to starve.

DOCTOR: It does seem hard to believe.

SECOND DOCTOR: Did you ever see practice so rotten? By the way, I was called over to your town about a week ago to see a kid I delivered up here during the summer. Do you know anything about the case?

DOCTOR: I probably got them on my list. Russians?

SECOND DOCTOR: Yeah, I thought as much. Has a job as a road worker or something. Said they couldn't pay me. Well, I took the trouble of going up to your courthouse and finding out what he makes. Eighteen dollars a week! And they had the nerve to tell me they couldn't pay me.

DOCTOR: She told me ten.

SECOND DOCTOR: She's a liar.

DOCTOR: Natural maternal instinct, I guess.

SECOND DOCTOR: Whiskey appetite, more like.

DOCTOR: Same thing.

SECOND DOCTOR: Okay, buddy. Only I'm telling you. And did I tell them. They'll never call me down there again, believe me. I had that much satisfaction out of them anyway. You make 'em pay you. Don't do anything for them unless they do. He's paid by the county. I tell you, if I had taxes to pay down there I'd go and take it out of his salary.

DOCTOR: You and how many others?

SECOND DOCTOR: They're bad actors, that crew. Do you know what they really do with their money? Whiskey. That old woman is the slickest customer you ever saw. Drunk all the time. Didn't you notice it?

DOCTOR: Not while I was there.

SECOND DOCTOR: Don't let them run the sympathy game on you. They tell me she leaves that baby lying on the bed all day long, screaming its head off until the neighbors complain to the police. The old skate's got nerves, you can see that. I can imagine she's a bugger when she gets going.

DOCTOR: But what about the young girl? She seems pretty straight.

SECOND DOCTOR: That thing! You mean the pimply-faced little bitch. If I had my way I'd run her out of town tomorrow morning. There's about a dozen wise guys on her tail every night of the week. Ask the cops. They know, but nobody will swear out a complaint. They say you'll stumble over her on the roof, behind the stairs, anytime at all. Boy, they sure took you in.

DOCTOR: Yeah, I suppose they did.

SECOND DOCTOR: But the old woman is the ringleader. She's got the brains. Take my advice and make them pay you.

[Second Doctor sits.]

NARRATOR: *[After a pause]* The last time I went I heard:

YOUNG GIRL: "Come in"

NARRATOR: from the front of the house. The fifteen-year-old was at the window, sitting in a rocking chair. She was holding the tightly wrapped baby in her arms. She got up.

[Young Girl stands.]

NARRATOR: Her legs were bare to the hips. A powerful little animal.

DOCTOR: What are you doing? Going swimming?

YOUNG GIRL: Nah, this is my gym suit. What the kids wear in gym class.

DOCTOR: How's the baby?

YOUNG GIRL: She's all right. She eats fine now.

DOCTOR: Good. *[Long, awkward pause]* Tell your mother to bring her to the office some day so I can weigh her. The food'll need increasing in a week or so anyway.

YOUNG GIRL: I'll tell her.

DOCTOR: Good. *[Awkward pause]* How's your face?

YOUNG GIRL: Gettin' better.

DOCTOR: My God, it *is*. Much better. *[Awkward pause]* Going back to school now?

YOUNG GIRL: Yeah. I had to.

END

QUESTIONS FOR DISCUSSION

What do you think of the physician in this story? What are his motivations for his interactions with the girl? Are there sexual overtones? Would he have helped her if he hadn't felt some attraction toward her? Does he act appropriately toward the mother? The baby? The girl? The story raises questions about what it is that motivates people to do the things they do. Are we sometimes selfish or self-indulgent when we do "good deeds"?

Who is the patient?

What would you have thought of the physician if the narrator had not told you the physician's unspoken thoughts? Does knowing the physician's thoughts change your view of him and his interactions with the girl?

At the very start of the story the physician expresses his negative attitude toward "foreigners." Is the family treated differently because they are foreigners? How does ethnicity play a role in the story? Do you think ethnicity plays a role in physician/patient encounters? Why is this story, written many years ago, not dated? How does it have relevance today?

Are the members of this family what you might characterize as difficult patients? Why? Do they deserve attentive medical care?

What kind of care did the baby receive in the hospital? Did the hospital staff miss the congenital heart defect diagnosis, or did the mother not want to let on to the physician that she knew about the child's heart problem?

Why is the mother so upset about the infant if she has six other healthy children? Why is this child her last hope?

Is the physician doing a good deed by caring for this indigent family?

What do you make of the physician's wife's reaction to the story her husband tells?

Why does the physician deny to the second physician in the locker room that the mother was drunk? Why does he return to the family for another visit when he knows he won't get paid?

What is the point of the dog discussion that the two physicians have?

Contrast the mother and the girl.

Where are your sympathies regarding the story's characters? How do you feel about the mother? The girl? The physician? The second physician? Given their situations in life, do any of the characters have or retain their dignity?

What do you think of the ending of the story?

Why is the story called "The Girl with a Pimply Face"? If the author had given the girl a name, would it have been as effective to title the story with the girl's name?

The Use of Force

WILLIAM CARLOS WILLIAMS

Adapted for Readers' Theater by Gregory A. Watkins

CAST
Narrator
Doctor
Mother
Father

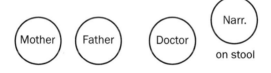

NOTES

This is a short script. The story is rich enough for a good discussion if performed alone, but may also be performed along with another story, for example, "Fetishes," which deals with a similar issue of physician versus patient control.

The person who takes the Narrator *part should be a strong, expressive reader.*

NARRATOR: They were new patients to me. All I had was the name: Olson.

MOTHER: Please come down as soon as you can. My daughter is very sick.

NARRATOR: When I arrived I was met by the mother, a big startled-looking woman, very clean and apologetic.

MOTHER: Is this the doctor? She's in the back. You must excuse us, Doctor, we have her in the kitchen where it is warm. It is very damp here sometimes.

NARRATOR: The child was fully dressed and sitting on her father's lap near the kitchen table. He tried to get up, but I motioned for him not to bother, took off my overcoat and started to look things over. I could see that they were all very nervous, eyeing me up and down distrustfully. As often in such cases, they weren't telling me more than they had to. It was up to me to tell them; that's why they were spending three dollars on me. The child was fairly eating me up with her cold, steady eyes, and no expression to her face whatever. She did not move and seemed, inwardly, quiet; an unusually attractive little thing, and as strong as a heifer in appearance. But her face was flushed, she was breathing rapidly, and I realized that she had a high fever. She had magnificent blonde hair, in profusion. One of those picture children often reproduced in advertising leaflets and the photogravure sections of the Sunday papers.

FATHER: She's had a fever for three days, and we don't know what it comes from. My wife has given her things, you know, like people do, but it don't do no good. And there's been a lot of sickness around. So we thought you'd better look her over and tell us what is the matter.

NARRATOR: As doctors often do I took a trial shot at it as a point of departure.

DOCTOR: Has she had a sore throat?

NARRATOR: Both parents answered me almost together . . .

FATHER: No . . . No, she says her throat don't hurt her.

MOTHER: Does your throat hurt you?

NARRATOR: The little girl's expression didn't change, nor did she move her eyes from my face.

DOCTOR: Have you looked?

MOTHER: I tried to, but I couldn't see.

NARRATOR: As it happens we had been having a number of cases of diphtheria during that month in the school to which this child went, and we were all, quite apparently, thinking of that, though no one had as yet spoken of the thing.

DOCTOR: Well, suppose we take a look at the throat first.

NARRATOR: I smiled in my best professional manner and asked for the child's first name.

MOTHER: Mathilda.

DOCTOR: Come on, Mathilda, open your mouth and let's take a look at your throat.

NARRATOR: Nothing doing.

DOCTOR: Aw, come on, just open your mouth wide and let me take a look. Look, I haven't anything in my hands. Just open up and let me see.

MOTHER: Such a nice man. Look how kind he is to you. Come on, do what he tells you to. He won't hurt you.

NARRATOR: At those words from the mother I ground my teeth in disgust. If only parents wouldn't use the word "hurt" I might be able to get somewhere. But I did not allow myself to be hurried or disturbed. Speaking quietly and slowly I approached the child again. As I moved my chair a little nearer, suddenly, with one catlike movement, both her hands clawed instinctively for my eyes. She almost reached them too. In fact, she knocked my glasses flying. They fell, though unbroken, several feet away from me on the kitchen floor.

MOTHER: You bad girl. Look what you've done. The nice man . . .

DOCTOR: For heaven's sake, Mrs. Olson. Don't call me a nice man to her. I'm here to look at her throat on the chance that she might have diphtheria and possibly die of it. But that's nothing to her.

Look here, Mathilda, we're going to look at your throat. You're old enough to understand what I'm saying. Will you open it now by yourself or shall we have to open it for you?

NARRATOR: Not a move. Even her expression hadn't changed. Her breaths, however, were coming faster and faster. Then the battle began. I had to do it. I had to have a throat culture for her protection. But first I told the parents:

DOCTOR: It's entirely up to you. It could be diphtheria and that's a dangerous disease. But I won't insist on a throat examination as long as you take the responsibility.

MOTHER: Mathilda, if you don't do what the doctor says you'll have to go to the hospital.

NARRATOR: Oh yeah? I had to smile to myself. After all, I had already fallen in love with the savage brat, though the parents were contemptible to me. In the ensuing struggle her parents grew more and more abject, crushed, exhausted, while the girl rose to magnificent heights of insane fury bred of her terror of me. The father tried his best, and he was a big man, but the fact that she was his daughter, his shame at her behavior, and his dread of hurting her made him release her just at the critical moment several times when I had almost achieved success, till I wanted to kill him. But his dread also that she might have diphtheria made him tell me to go on, go on though he himself was almost fainting, while the mother moved back and forth behind us raising and lowering her hands in an agony of apprehension.

DOCTOR: Mr. Olson, put her in front of you on your lap, and hold both her wrists.

NARRATOR: But as soon as he did the child let out a scream: "Don't," she cried. "You're hurting me. Let go of my hands. Let them go, I tell you. Stop it! Stop it! You're killing me!"

MOTHER: *[Very upset]* Doctor, do you think she can stand it?

FATHER: *[Frustrated, angry]* You get out, Mother. Do you want her to die of diphtheria?

DOCTOR: Come on now, hold her.

NARRATOR: Then I grasped the child's head with my left hand and tried to get the wooden tongue depressor between her teeth. She fought, with clenched teeth, desperately. But now I also had grown furious — at a child. I tried to hold myself down but I couldn't. I know how to expose a throat for inspection, and I did my best. When I finally got the wooden spatula behind her front teeth and just the point of it into the mouth cavity, she opened up for an instant. Before I could see anything, she bit down again and, gripping the wooden blade between her molars, she reduced it to splinters before I could get it out again.

MOTHER: Mathilda, aren't you ashamed? Aren't you ashamed to act like that in front of the doctor?

DOCTOR: *[Desperate]* Get me a smooth-handled spoon of some sort. We're going through with this.

NARRATOR: The child's mouth was already bleeding. Her tongue was cut and she was screaming in wild hysterical shrieks. Perhaps I should have desisted and come back in an hour or more. No doubt it would have been better. But I had seen at least two children lying dead in bed of neglect in such cases, and, feeling that I must get a diagnosis now or never, I went at it again. The worst of it was that I, too, had got beyond reason. I could have torn the child apart in my own fury and enjoyed it. It was a pleasure to attack her. My face was burning with it. The damned little brat must be protected against her own idiocy, and others must be protected against her. It is social necessity. All these things are true. But in a blind fury, a feeling of adult shame, bred of a longing for muscular release, I overpowered the child's neck and jaws. I forced the heavy silver spoon back of her teeth and down her throat till she gagged. And there it was — both tonsils covered with membrane. She had fought valiantly to keep me from knowing her secret. She had been hiding that sore throat for three days at least and lying to her parents in order to escape just such an outcome as this. Now, truly, she was furious. She had been on the defensive before, but now she attacked. Tried to get off her father's lap and fly at me while tears of defeat blinded her eyes.

END

QUESTIONS FOR DISCUSSION

Why was the physician so determined to get a throat culture?

Was the physician justified in using force to obtain the culture?

How would you have handled the situation if you were the physician? The parents?

What point do you think the author of the story is trying to make?

Why were the parents contemptible to the physician?

What was your reaction to each of the characters in the story?

Is there a culture or class difference issue lurking in this story? What is your evidence?

Why did the physician feel "adult shame" at forcing Mathilda to open her mouth for the culture? Why, despite this feeling, did the physician persist? What was wrong with the physician's actions?

What does it mean that the physician had "fallen in love with the savage brat"? What do you make of the sexual innuendoes and imagery the author uses? Was this a sexual attack?

Is it acceptable for physicians or other health care providers to have positive and negative feelings about their patients? Did the physician in the story cross a line and act on his feelings, or was he doing what was necessary to protect the girl and the community?

Fetishes

RICHARD SELZER

Adapted for Readers' Theater by Gregory A. Watkins

CAST

Narrator

Audrey

Leonard

Violet

Surgeon

Dowling

Bhimjee

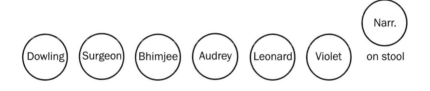

NOTES

"Fetishes" and "A Use of Force" can be performed as part of the same program, as they raise similar issues. One person can read both Surgeon *and* Dowling *if desired. The person who reads* Bhimjee *could, with good effect, use an Indian accent.*

NARRATOR: Audrey had waited until she was thirty-two to marry. Not by choice; no one had asked her. But all the time she had never given up hope. So, when Leonard Blakeslee had come along, she had at once reached out her hands for him as though he were an exotic foreign dish whose very strangeness captured her appetite completely.

AUDREY: You'll love me?

NARRATOR: And never once in all the years since had he given her reason to doubt it. The fact that no children had come along was briefly regretted by both of them, then accepted. Somehow, it suited them. Leonard is an anthropologist. Every so often he goes off to New Guinea on an expedition among the Asmat. It's the only time they're separated. When he's away, Audrey feels only half intact, bisected. And Leonard too, as he wrote in a letter (Audrey has saved them all) . . .

LEONARD: I am never done with wanting you at my side, where you ought always to be, my darling.

NARRATOR: She loved that "ought always to be."

AUDREY: It is courtly.

NARRATOR: When he's not going on in that vein, his letters are anthropological, having to do with the language of the tribe for which he is compiling a dictionary, the artifacts he is collecting, the myths and mores of the people, all of which Audrey reads with affection and even genuine interest.

AUDREY: [Smiling] Leonard and his artifacts.

NARRATOR: Not that Audrey is beautiful. No one but Leonard could accuse her of that. But what she had, she had, and that was the true love of her husband. Another thing Audrey has right now is a ten-centimeter cyst on her right ovary that the doctors can't say for certain is benign, and so it will have to come out.

AUDREY: Thank heavens Leonard isn't off on one of his expeditions.

NARRATOR: Fifteen years ago (she had been forty-two then), every one of her upper teeth had been extracted while Leonard was in New Guinea. "Pyorrhea," the dentist had said. "You've let it go. They are all rotten and ready to fall out on their own."

AUDREY: [Flabbergasted] I have to think. My husband isn't here. He's in New Guinea.

NARRATOR: She would remember the dentist's contemptuous little smile. On the way home, she said to her sister, Violet . . .

AUDREY: But . . . Leonard . . .

VIOLET: Leonard is not a dentist.

NARRATOR: And so, a few days later, Audrey had gone through with it. She hadn't been out of the dentist's office ten minutes when she knew that she had made a dreadful mistake. Violet drove her home afterward. Lying down on the back seat of the car, her mouth numb, her cheeks stuffed with pledgets of cotton, she wondered what Leonard would think, how he would feel. And she recalled something she had heard him say to one of his students, she couldn't remember why.

LEONARD: No one can take your dignity away from you; you might throw it away yourself, but no one can take it away from you.

NARRATOR: Then and there Audrey decided that Leonard didn't have to know.

VIOLET: You all right?

NARRATOR: Right from the start, Audrey refused to take the denture out of her mouth, no matter the pain. There were dark blisters on her gums; she lisped. But she was determined. Leonard would be coming home in two months. Audrey persevered so that with weeks to spare, she had gotten used to the "prosthesis," as they called it, incorporated it. It had become second nature. Oh, she had to steel herself against the first times it had to come out, be cleaned, then reinserted. But she had surprised herself. She was calm, curious even, as she turned it over in her hand, examining. Like a pink horseshoe, she decided, and how wise she was to have avoided the vulgarity of pure white. Ivory was more natural. Ivory has endured; ivory has kept faith. In time her palate had molded itself to fit, her gums were snug and secure in the hollow trough. Never, never would she remove her teeth anywhere but in a locked bathroom. She would keep them in at night. It was a myth that you had to take your dentures out at night. Before long, she had no qualms, didn't mind at all. The denture had become for her a kind of emblem of personal dignity, like one of those Asmat artifacts with magic properties, but this having to do with the one thing that mattered most to Audrey: Leonard.

AUDREY: It isn't really cheating.

VIOLET: You're lucky. You're one of those people who don't show their teeth when they smile.

NARRATOR: When at last Leonard burst into the room, gathered her in his arms and kissed her, she smiled as much from triumph as with happiness.

LEONARD: You never cease to charm me.

NARRATOR: And she knew then that she had done it. Leonard would never know. But now it was fifteen years later. And the surgeon was saying:

SURGEON: *[He takes himself very seriously.]* Total abdominal hysterectomy. A clean sweep.

AUDREY: What does that include?

SURGEON: The uterus, both ovaries, both tubes.

AUDREY: Why my uterus? Why my left ovary? My tubes?

NARRATOR: He then explained, rather too patiently, she thought, that she didn't need her reproductive organs anymore.

SURGEON: The risk of getting cancer in one of those organs is not inconsiderable.

AUDREY: Human beings don't talk like that,

NARRATOR: she thought.

AUDREY: That is not human speech.

SURGEON: And, as long as we're going to be in there anyway . . .

AUDREY: In there!

NARRATOR: Audrey couldn't keep her hand from passing lightly across her abdomen. Then he spoke about the small additional risk of the larger operation, said it was "negligible." But Audrey already knew what it was to go through life missing something. She wished fervently she had been able to keep her cyst a secret, like her teeth. You would think it would be easier since the ovaries were inside and safely hidden. Imagine having to carry them in a bag between your legs, like testicles. And as for the risk of getting cancer . . . is that a reason to have your organs taken out?

AUDREY: All of life is a risk. Living in California is a risk; there might be an earthquake.

NARRATOR: First, her teeth, and now her . . . her womanhood, yes it was nothing short of that. All at once the operation seemed part of a plot to take her body apart. And she remembered the clink of coins years ago, as that dentist stirred the change in his pocket, stirred it on and on, enjoying the sound of it before he took up the syringe and injected her with novocaine. On the wall in back of the surgeon's desk was a colored diagram of the female organs. Altogether, it resembled a sweet-faced cow's head rising to the gentle curve of the horns.

AUDREY: No. No, that cannot be. Only my ovary, the one with the cyst. Nothing else, unless there is cancer.

NARRATOR: She would sign permission only for that. But in the end, she capitulated.

SURGEON: You're doing the right thing, I assure you, Mrs. Blakeslee.

NARRATOR: At the hospital, Leonard and Audrey followed the nurse into the room. The nurse held up a knee-length shirt open at the back. "Get undressed and into this," the nurse said. Audrey did and over it put on the pale green brocade bed jacket Leonard had given her the night before. It had been arranged that Leonard was to wait in the solarium outside the rooms. The surgeon would talk to him there, let him know what he had found. Afterward, he would wait for Audrey to be wheeled down from the recovery room a few hours later.

LEONARD: Good luck.

NARRATOR: He's frightened, she thought, and felt tears filming her eyes. After Leonard had left, Audrey lay on the bed, thinking of him — the silky feel of the black hairs on his forearms, his smell of permanence, the sound of his singing. Leonard sang bass. It was her favorite. At sixty-one, his voice was as rich as ever. Sometimes, listening in church to that submarine vibrato, she would have moments of unecclesiastical commotion. Once, when she confessed it, Leonard reproached her with a waggle of his finger. Ah, but his was a magic throat.

DOWLING: *[Dowling stands.]* *[Always stern, humorless, and pompous]* I'm Dr. Dowling.

NARRATOR: The man had knocked and come in at the same time. It is what happens in hospitals, Audrey thought. She was glad to be wearing the green bed jacket. So long as she had it on, there was protection.

DOWLING: I'm the anesthesiologist. I'll be putting you to sleep tomorrow. Any questions?

NARRATOR: Audrey shook her head. He had an important sort of face, florid, with jowls made even more congressional by the white political hair that escaped from beneath his green surgical cap. He was wearing a scrub suit of the same color and, over that, a white laboratory coat. The strings of a mask dangled.

DOWLING: Open your mouth as wide as you can. *[Pause]* I see you have an upper plate. Out it comes in the morning before you leave this room. The nurse will mind it for you.

AUDREY: *[Frightened]* But I never take it out, only to clean . . .

DOWLING: Well, you can't go to the operating room with it in. I can't put you to sleep with a foreign body in your mouth.

AUDREY: Foreign body!

NARRATOR: Audrey felt the blood leave her head. Gongs could not have sounded louder in her ears. Then a final cold ticking.

AUDREY: For how long . . . ?

DOWLING: Until you're fully awake. Certainly till evening.

AUDREY: But you don't understand . . .

NARRATOR: she began. Her voice trailed off. The doctor waited, turned his head, looked at her from a corner of his eye.

DOWLING: Yes?

AUDREY: It is . . . my husband does not know that I have a denture. He has been unaware of it for fifteen years. I would not want him to see me without it. *[Quietly]* Please, it is important to me.

DOWLING: Pride. No room for it here. Like modesty. Suppose we had to get at your trachea, your windpipe, in a hurry, and then we had to waste time fishing those teeth out. Suppose they came loose in the middle of the operation. There are a hundred supposes.

NARRATOR: He started to go.

AUDREY: It isn't pride.

DOWLING: What, then?

AUDREY: It's dignity.

NARRATOR: Perhaps it had been pride at the very beginning, but it had grown. And something else: Audrey understood that the connubial apparatus of a man is more delicate than a woman's. She saw no need to put it to the test.

DOWLING: Come now, Mrs. Blakeslee, is it really dignity? You're making too much of it.

NARRATOR: All right, then, she would calculate, be a cat.

AUDREY: Don't you . . . don't you have a little something hidden away that you wouldn't want anyone to know about?

DOWLING: *[Hesitates]* No, actually not.

AUDREY: How boring. And, of course, I don't for a minute believe you.

NARRATOR: This doctor could not know it, but Audrey was fighting for her life. But now she saw that he had retreated a vast safe distance behind his lips.

DOWLING: In any case, you may not keep them in. And that's that.

NARRATOR: He stood abruptly and walked to the door.

DOWLING: Have a good night. *[Dowling sits.]*

NARRATOR: After he had left, Audrey felt her heart go small in her chest. Again there was the clink of coins being stirred in a pocket. With a sudden resolve, she decided that there was no longer any need for tact. The situation didn't call for tact. It called for defiance.

AUDREY: I'll sign myself out of the hospital. Against medical advice, as they say. That cyst might well be benign. They don't know. Leaving it in would be just one more risk.

NARRATOR: A risk infinitely smaller than having Leonard see her without her denture. Her mouth caved in, wrinkled like a drawstring pouch. She tried to imagine herself saying to Leonard afterward . . .

AUDREY: All right, then. You have seen what you have seen. Now accept it. Or not.

NARRATOR: But she couldn't. That way lay death. Hers or that of something far more delicate and valuable. No, she thought. No. Never again would she cultivate a belief in invulnerability. Audrey reached for the telephone, dialed.

AUDREY: Leonard, don't come to the hospital at all tomorrow.

LEONARD: But why? Of course I'm coming to see you.

AUDREY: That's just the point, Leonard. Please . . . please. Don't come. Promise me.

LEONARD: I'm sorry, Audrey. I'm just not going to agree to that. So forget it.

AUDREY: I don't want you to see me like that.

LEONARD: *[Smiling]* Like what? I have seen it all before, you know.

NARRATOR: Oh, but you haven't, she thought. You shouldn't.

LEONARD: What is it, Audrey? You sound distraught. Shall I come right over? I'll make them let me in.

AUDREY: *[Harshly]* I just wanted to spare you. There are times when people need to be alone.

LEONARD: No. I'll be there.

NARRATOR: *[Pause]* Violet managed the gift shop in the lobby of the hospital. She was two years older than Audrey — a big woman, divorced once, widowed once. Violet did not use makeup.

VIOLET: I have nothing to hide.

NARRATOR: Still, she dyed her hair. For business reasons.

VIOLET: When you have to meet the public, gray hair automatically dismisses you.

NARRATOR: Fifteen years before, they had been closer, when Violet had brought Audrey home from the dentist's office and Audrey had sworn her sister to a lifetime of silence. But somewhere between then and now Vi had become the kind of woman who sat herself down with ceremony in a deep chair to receive the secrets of others. She would be coming up to the room after she closed the gift shop. Audrey would ask for a ride home. She would deal with Leonard later.

VIOLET: I'll do no such thing. Do you mean to lie there and tell me that Leonard still doesn't know about your false teeth?

NARRATOR: Vi made a point of never saying "denture." "False teeth" had a balder sound and they had drifted too far apart for softness. The venules on Vi's cheeks dilated with indignant blood. Audrey reached for the light switch, flicked it off. It was something to do.

AUDREY: May I turn off the light?

VIOLET: Listen, Audrey, this has become a sick obsession with you.

AUDREY: There are madder things.

NARRATOR: And she lamented the weakness that made her let down her guard before this stranger who was her sister.

VIOLET: Besides, it's a lie. People shouldn't lie, whatever.

AUDREY: Oh, lies. That's where you're wrong. People don't lie enough. When people tell the whole truth, that's when things fall apart. Most relationships are like some plants, I think. They need to be kept partly in the shade or they wither.

NARRATOR: A nurse came in and turned on the light. In the sudden glare Violet leaped up at her.

VIOLET: Now, Audrey, don't be stupid. Behave yourself.

NARRATOR: Violet's teeth would never fall out, Audrey thought. They chew words, worry them; the way they buckle up her mouth. Almost at once there was a hesitant knock at the door.

AUDREY: Oh, God. Now what?

BHIMJEE: *[Stands]* My name is Dr. Bhimjee. I am the intern on this ward.

NARRATOR: An Indian or Pakistani, she thought. And lame. He limped toward the bed using his head and one arm in the act of locomotion.

BHIMJEE: Mrs. Blakeslee, I see that both our names end with two e's.

NARRATOR: His face was dark, she suspected, more from fatigue than from racial coloring. More than anything else he resembled an ungainly parcel, something bulgy and ill-wrapped. His hair was almost too thick, too black, but relieved by a single swatch of white near the crown. He is not young, Audrey decided. What has he endured and with how much patience? All at once, a fence came down. Who, after all, is to say where, in whom, one places trust?

AUDREY: I have false teeth.

NARRATOR: She was shocked at the ease with which the forbidden words had come. The intern gazed down at her.

BHIMJEE: Many people do.

NARRATOR: The slate-colored skin set off the perfection of his own very white teeth. He is beautiful, she thought. And she threw herself further upon his mercy.

AUDREY: I have had them for fifteen years. My husband has never seen me without them. He doesn't know that I have them. The anesthetist was here. He says I must leave them here in the room tomorrow. My husband will be waiting for me to come back from the recovery room. He will see me. I can't do that. Please, please.

NARRATOR: For a long moment they looked at each other, during which something, a covenant perhaps, Audrey didn't know, was exchanged. A rush of profound affection came over her. It was nothing like her feeling for Leonard, but for all she knew, it might have been love.

BHIMJEE: Do not worry. In the morning, put them in the nightstand. There is a container. I will take them with me to the operation. I am assigned to your case, so I will be there too. Before you leave the recovery room, I will put them back into your mouth. Do not worry.

NARRATOR: Later, when she awoke in the recovery room, the pain of her incision was the *second* thing Audrey felt. The first was the denture, which she explored with her tongue. Only then came the pain that, so help her, she didn't mind. In spite of it, she curled up like a cat in a basket. Once, when she opened her eyes, she saw, or thought she saw, a dark face above her, a white swatch in a tumble of black hair, like a plume of smoke clinging to the chimney of a snug cottage.

BHIMJEE: Don't worry. Your teeth are in. Take a deep breath. *[Pause]* Again.

NARRATOR: He checked her pulse, and was gone.

[Bhimjee sits.]

For a long time his voice lingered, lapsing, returning, drifting into darkness. And then there was Leonard, holding her hand, leaning over the bed to kiss her.

LEONARD: The doctor says it was benign.

NARRATOR: During the days that followed, Audrey found herself thinking about Dr. Bhimjee as much as she did about Leonard. There was a peacefulness about him. Not resignation so much as acceptance. No, definitely not resignation. Resignation suggests defeat. Acceptance, rather. Where had he found it? Wrestled it, she supposed, barehanded from a tangle of thorns. He had no need to deceive. It had not been given him to deceive. She saw him differently now from the way she had that first desperate night. What she had thought was fatigue became the sum total of all the suffering he had experienced. It had worn his face down to the bone. The sockets of his eyes were dark cabins of it. Audrey would have liked to take the bony parcel in her arms, to breathe in his dreams. *[Pause]*

And soon it was the hour of Audrey's discharge from the hospital. The intern had come to say good-bye. *[Bhimjee stands.]*

LEONARD: My wife tells me you have been very kind to her.

BHIMJEE: Not at all.

LEONARD: I want you to know that I will always remember your *[struggles]* . . . your courtesy.

BHIMJEE: Please, it was nothing.

LEONARD: Nevertheless. Nevertheless, I want you to have this.

NARRATOR: He held out a small reddish stone.

BHIMJEE: What is that?

LEONARD: Just a stone that has been dyed red by the Asmat people of New Guinea. See? It has a monkey carved on one side, a parrot on the other. A shaman gave it to me. He's sort of a doctor too. It wards off melancholy, brings good luck. Please, take it.

NARRATOR: The doctor hesitated.

LEONARD: I want you to have it.

NARRATOR: Maybe it was the sun probing between the slats of the venetian blinds, but from her perspective it seemed to Audrey that, at the exact moment when the red stone left the white hand of one and entered the dark hand of the other, something flared up that looked for all the world like fire.

END

QUESTIONS FOR DISCUSSION

The discussion leader might want to bring along a dictionary definition of the word "fetish" to use during the discussion.

Was Audrey's request reasonable? What does her sister Violet think? What is Violet's role in the story?

Can you justify the anesthesiologist's response to Audrey's request?

Is the denture issue a matter of pride, as the anesthesiologist states, or of dignity, as Audrey thinks? Why not just tell Leonard the truth? Why is this denture matter such an issue for Audrey?

Does Audrey retain her dignity?

Why does Dr. Bhimjee help Audrey when other physicians wouldn't or couldn't? Is there something special about him that makes him more likely to help someone in Audrey's situation? Does his "otherness" (limp, foreignness, age, skin color, accent) play a role in the story? Does "otherness" play a role in the way medicine is practiced today?

Have you had experiences like Audrey's? *or* As a caregiver, have you been in a situation where circumstances like Audrey's arose? How did you respond?

What does Audrey feel toward Bhimjee?

To what does the title of the story refer? Why is the word in the title plural rather than singular?

Do you think Leonard really knows Audrey's secret? What is your evidence?

What do you make of the last lines of the story?

What are the connections between this story and "The Use of Force"?

PART II. BEING A PHYSICIAN

◉ ◉ ◉ ◉ ◉

Ambulance

SUSAN ONTHANK MATES

Adapted for Readers' Theater by Gregory A. Watkins

CAST
Student

Narrator

Marie

Operator

Guard

Intern

Chief Resident (Chief)

Driver

ER Nurse

Aide

Admitting Clerk (Clerk)

Head Nurse (Head)

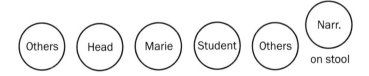

NOTES

"Laundry" and "Ambulance" can be performed in the same program. They both deal with the human side of being a physician or a physician-in-training.

The minor roles may be played by two or three readers using a different voice for each character. Possible configurations are (1) Operator/Aide, Chief Resident/Guard/Driver, *and* Admitting Clerk/ER Nurse/Intern; *(2)* Operator/Intern/ER Nurse/Clerk *and* Guard/Chief Resident/Driver/Aide. *Also,* Marie *and* Head Nurse *could be played by the same person.* Marie *and* Head Nurse *are black women and* Student *is a white woman, though in a readers' theater performance like this the readers need not match those descriptions since the context of the story conveys that information.*

STUDENT: I think I'll put my feet up with you, Marie.

NARRATOR: Marie was a practical nurse working the evening shift at the old Lincoln Hospital in the South Bronx. The city only paid for registered nurses on the day shift. Not that the patients weren't in completely capable hands with Marie. She was a sharp Jamaican dust-storm of a woman — tiny, wiry, and astoundingly energetic. Most evenings, the ward hopped like a nightclub with one demented act; she sang, she scolded, she exhorted, she divulged. She was an efficient pied piper, sucking those sick people right out of themselves, away from broken linoleum and army-green cloth partitions and the disinfected stench of the open ward. On Marie's shift, the junkies were so entertained they even gave up their usual pastime of knocking the roaches off the curtains.

STUDENT: Pretty quiet on the ward tonight, Marie.

MARIE: Yup. Chores are done, everyone's tucked in. We can rest our feet for a little while.

NARRATOR: I was sweating in the heat of the New York night, but she was starchy and crisp as usual. Marie's voice was as quick and precise as her body, accompanied by the whirr of the fan, the flies buzzing, and the chanting. Always the chanting.

MARIE: I call them my singers, the ones who go to their death not groaning, not screaming, but singing, coaxing death with a chant of "gates, gates, gates in the sky," or "wash the baby, the baby, Oh Lord, the baby," or "cooking, scrubbing, cooking, scrubbing."

NARRATOR: The three old women chanters were placed one on each end of the ward and one in the middle. Marie always prepared them for the night by smoothing their pillows and straightening their sheets, as if they were still aware. And they just kept on crooning their way into death, putting the rest of us to sleep. *[Pause]* Marie started talking to me about her son.

MARIE: That one, my Jamey, he's a smart one. He put himself in law school, oh my. He's gonna be something. He always was a crackerjack.

STUDENT: Is he married?

MARIE: Oh, sure, and the first little one on the way. Imagine me a grandmama.

STUDENT: Marie, don't you have another son?

MARIE: Yeah honey, I do.

STUDENT: What does he do?

MARIE: I don't know. I haven't seen him now, two years it will be. I lost him young.

NARRATOR: She sat absolutely still.

STUDENT: Lost him to what, if you don't mind my asking?

MARIE: Lost him to the streets. *[Changing the subject]* Jamey, though, now you should have seen him in high school. Wasn't he the sharp one!

NARRATOR: I didn't ask anymore about the other son. *[Pause]* In that silence, the paging began.

It started innocently. First . . .

OPERATOR: *[Always in a nasal voice]* ER Chief to the emergency room.

NARRATOR: Nothing much to wonder about. Then . . .

OPERATOR: Security personnel to the emergency room.

NARRATOR: And then . . .

OPERATOR: All senior doctors to the emergency room.

NARRATOR: Finally . . .

OPERATOR: All doctors to the ER stat, all doctors to the ER stat.

NARRATOR: I jumped off my chair and looked at Marie.

MARIE: Not you, honey, you're a medical student.

STUDENT: But what's going on down there?

MARIE: Whatever it is, you best stay here. You'll be the only kind of doctor we got up here now.

OPERATOR: All medical students to the emergency room, stat, all medical students to the emergency room, stat.

NARRATOR: *[Animated and excited]* This time I tore down the hall, my short white coat flying. There was no safe place to leave things at Lincoln, so when you came for overnight duty, you brought everything in your pockets. Coins, notebooks, ophthalmoscope, pens, syringes, and Tampax came jumping out of my pockets as I rounded the stairwell. I clutched my pockets and tried to glide. As I came down the last hall, I could hear the emergency room — yells and screams and a general chaotic chorus. I charged into the waiting room and stopped dead. Wooden chairs had been overturned. The middle of the room was a twitching mass of muscle and skin, with a pause provided here and there by a knife blade, a chain, an ice pick. I had seen knife fights in the waiting room before, but the scale of this one was staggering. Kids in studded leather jackets going at each other. One boy's jacket had "Death Lords" spelled across the back. On the floor were two clumps of doctors and nurses trying to resuscitate bleeding bodies. The audience to all this was the arriving relatives and girlfriends, some in torn jeans, some in cheap businesslike suits, some dressed for a night on the town. They were crying and reaching from the sidelines. I stood paralyzed by the entrance. One of the guards spotted me there:

GUARD: *[In a typical New York accent]* G'won through to the treatment area!

NARRATOR: Without thinking, I plunged through the spectacle and found myself in the treatment area. Here things were much the same, except there were more bodies lying flat with people working on them, and fewer still upright, causing damage. A surgical intern grabbed me:

INTERN: Put your hand here on this man's neck to stop the bleeding.

NARRATOR: I did as told, but as I stepped closer, I let the pressure slack a second and a hot shower of blood sprayed over me, soaking into my whites, splattering my face. I pushed harder and it stopped. Then an arm brushed my shoulder. I turned with a jump to see the Chief Resident on duty that night. He was shouting something at me. I grabbed a nearby hand and pressed it on the neck wound, then followed the Chief Resident.

CHIEF: Medical student?

STUDENT: Yes, sir.

CHIEF: Need you to ride an ambulance. Supposed to send an M.D., but we can't spare any. You'll have to go. Go out to the bay, we'll bring the patient.

NARRATOR: The night air was a shock — dark, cool, and quiet. An ambulance sat there, back doors open, ready to receive. The driver leaned out, an unremarkable man. He pulled the pipe out of his mouth.

DRIVER: You the doc?

STUDENT: Yes.

NARRATOR: He nodded contentedly and disappeared again into the dark.

CHIEF: Hey, medical student!

NARRATOR: A nurse and an orderly were wheeling out a stretcher. A still form lay on it, gleaming in the night. I ran over.

CHIEF: Here's the papers. You'll have to bag him.

NARRATOR: He handed me the bag. I had never used one before. I squeezed it as he had, forcing the air down the tube into the lungs. He turned to walk away.

STUDENT: But where are we going? What am I supposed to do?

CHIEF: Keep him alive if you can. Gotta get back to the ER.

NARRATOR: The nurse and the orderly lifted the stretcher into the ambulance and rolled the patient onto the narrow cot attached to one side. I was moving with them, trying to squeeze the bag in a kind of breathing-dance. I had never paid much attention to breathing before. They closed the doors of the ambulance and I was alone in the dimly lit back. The frail papers of the temporary chart were barely readable.

STUDENT: [To herself] What does this say? "Transport unknown male to Jacobi Hospital for neurosurgery. Bullet wound to head."

NARRATOR: I looked down at him. He was eighteen or twenty, motionless aside from my breathing for him. His face was serene, as if lost in the deep sleep of childhood. The top of his head was bandaged, but there was no other mark on the smooth skin of his body.

STUDENT: [To herself] I wonder what his name is?

NARRATOR: The ambulance started, the siren went on with a deafening wail, and we shot out of the hospital bay. The violence of the ride surprised me; I was barely able to keep my balance as we swerved through the dense traffic.

STUDENT: [To herself] Keep squeezing the bag. Keep squeezing the bag . . .

NARRATOR: I kept telling myself. But I was frightened. The light inside the ambulance flickered with each maneuver, as if with a faulty connection. Then disaster struck. A car cut in front of us. The ambulance driver veered suddenly. I went flying and landed with a crack against the glass of the rear doors. I turned to look for the boy. (I called him Angelo.)

STUDENT: Damn!

NARRATOR: He had slid off his cot and onto the floor, and was turning dusky blue.

STUDENT: *[Yelling]* Driver!!

NARRATOR: But nothing could be heard over the noise of the siren. Panicked, I straightened his body and smoothed the pillow under his head. I forced a sudden, rational calm.

STUDENT: *[To herself]* Think. Reason this out. He's turning blue because he doesn't have enough air. Give him air.

NARRATOR: I tried to squeeze the bag harder. Nothing moved. So . . .

STUDENT: *[To herself]* The tube is blocked.

NARRATOR: I looked at the tube. It had been pulled out when he fell, and the end was stuck in his mouth.

STUDENT: *[To herself]* If the tube isn't in the lungs, the air isn't going there. How am I going to get air to his lungs? Oh Angelo, stay alive. Mouth-to-mouth resuscitation. I'll just keep it up 'til we get there.

NARRATOR: I yanked the tube completely out and pulled back his jaw. We were still sliding back and forth across the floor of the ambulance as it jerked and turned, accelerated and stopped.

STUDENT: *[To herself]* OK. I learned this. I can do this.

NARRATOR: I did it. I didn't notice that we were there until they opened the back doors, flooding the ambulance with the neon lights of Jacobi's emergency room. The light hurt my eyes, but I didn't dare stop breathing. I just stayed where I was, breathing into Angelo's mouth . . . and, a minute later, an ER nurse tore me away from him.

ER NURSE: My, what a picture you look!

NARRATOR: She pulled me out of the ambulance.

ER NURSE: We hear you had a real gang war down there at Lincoln!

STUDENT: Yes.

NARRATOR: I was still dazed. My mouth was coming out of numbness into bruised stinging. I touched my tongue to my lips, feeling their swollen strangeness. Angelo was being taken off by the trauma team.

ER NURSE: Why don't you go get a cup of coffee. Bobby here will wait for you, won't you, Bobby?

NARRATOR: She looked up at the driver. He nodded calmly, pulling on his pipe.

DRIVER: Sure.

NARRATOR: I went in. Some of my medical student friends assigned to Jacobi drifted around me, trapped by my bloodied whites like small animals frozen in the headlights of an oncoming car. They made nonchalant conversation about trauma and gang war and other things we didn't understand. I barely heard them, the roaring darkness filling my ears as if I had crossed from another world and wasn't quite back into this one. When I tried to go to the cafeteria, one of the aides stopped me.

AIDE: *[Standing]* You look disgusting with all that blood all over you. You can't go round people like that.

NARRATOR: I looked at him.

STUDENT: I need a cup of coffee. I have no change of clothes with me.

NARRATOR: But in the well-lit hospital corridor, I knew I was inappropriate, wearing so much blood. *[Aide sits.]* I went back out to the ambulance and climbed in the front. The driver looked at me.

DRIVER: Got some coffee?

STUDENT: No.

DRIVER: Ah, people are like that.

NARRATOR: We rode back quietly, *smoothly*. When we pulled up to Lincoln Hospital, he said:

DRIVER: Got another call. I'll just let you off.

NARRATOR: I slid off the seat and jumped to the ground.

STUDENT: Thanks. *[Pause]* Doesn't it bother you, ferrying people back and forth, night after night?

NARRATOR: He must not have heard me, because he didn't answer. The ambulance took off, leaving me standing there alone. *[Pause]* The next morning I stopped by Jacobi on the way to Lincoln. There was no sign of "unknown male" on the neurosurgical ward or in the recovery room. I asked the clerk at the admitting office.

CLERK: Nope. Can't find him listed anywhere. Usually, when they disappear like that, it means they died before they could get properly admitted.

NARRATOR: When I got to Lincoln, the head nurse on days stopped me in the hall. She was an old friend of Marie's.

HEAD: *[Stands up]* So I hear you rode the ambulance last night.

NARRATOR: She was a̶ ̶l̶a̶r̶g̶e̶ an imperious woman, and she looked down at me without smiling.

STUDENT: Yes.

HEAD: Folks at Jacobi tell me you were giving that boy mouth-to-mouth when you got there. That's a good way to get all sorts of disease.

NARRATOR: She paused for a minute, as if she were going to say something more, then turned to go.

HEAD: Remind me to teach you how to use the ambubag sometime.

NARRATOR: Something of what I was feeling must have shown on my face, because she suddenly frowned and grabbed me by the shoulders.

HEAD: *[Firmly, angrily]* Do you think you should have saved him? Who do you think you are? Better that you tried to save that boy's life, not just in one minute in the end, but year after year after year, and you some white girl gonna come down here and make everything all right in a few minutes?

NARRATOR: She was trembling now. She pushed by me and ran down the hall. *[Head Nurse sits.]*

I saw Marie later that night. She was smoothing down the pillow for one of the chanters, the one with breast cancer. The old woman was out of her mind and didn't notice, but Marie was smoothing her pillow and pulling up her blanket anyway. I walked up to her.

STUDENT: Anything else you need before I go to dinner?

MARIE: I heard about you riding the ambulance with that boy that got shot.

STUDENT: Yeah, well I didn't do much for him, did I?

NARRATOR: I tried to turn away before she could say anything more, but she was too fast for me. She fumbled in her pocket and pulled out some dog-eared Polaroids.

MARIE: Here, let me show you something. My new grandbaby, just born last night. Isn't she beautiful?

NARRATOR: She smiled like the moon breaking loose on a cloudy night.

END

QUESTIONS FOR DISCUSSION

What did the medical student learn from her experience?

Why was the head nurse so upset with the student at the end? Was she justified? In what ways are race and ethnicity integral parts of the message of this story? Is medicine's role to deal with the larger issues of society or with the narrower matter of healing the sick?

Did the medical student do something wrong in trying to save the teenage boy? Why does she try to save his life? Was she trying to be a hero? Was his minority status of significance to her in the actions she took? How does she deal with this young man's death?

Is the student's gender of importance to the story? Might the story have unfolded differently had the student been a male? If so, why and how?

What do you make of Marie? How does she handle the dying patients on her floor? How does she handle the loss of one of her sons? What is the significance of the birth of her grandchild?

What do you learn about medical students from this story? About nurses?

Laundry

SUSAN ONTHANK MATES

Adapted for Readers' Theater by Gregory A. Watkins

CAST

Protagonist as Mother (Mother)

Protagonist as Doctor (Doctor)

Protagonist as Person (Person)

Mr. Dantio (Dantio)

Surgeon (Surgeon)

Mrs. Dantio (Mrs. D)

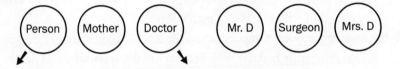

[arrows show seating and eye-focus angle]

NOTES

"Laundry" and "Ambulance" can be performed in the same program. They both deal with the human side of being a physician or a physician-in-training.

The discussion leader should announce before the performance that the adapter, Greg Watkins, divided the protagonist of the story into three separate roles in the readers' theater script to accentuate the portrayal of the mother, physician, and human being in her. Mother *and* Person *reflect only the thoughts, feelings, and memories of the protagonist, while* Doctor *actually interacts with the characters in the story.* Mother, *sitting between* Person *and* Doctor, *should keep her eyes focused straight out over the audience to the back of the room.* Person *and*

Doctor *should sit at angles to* Mother *and keep their eyes focused in the direction in which they are sitting — offstage right or left.*

MOTHER: *[Recalling]* I was folding the baby's diapers — cloth, the kind they make now with a double thickness down the middle — and the phone rang. I was thinking and not thinking; just a second before, the baby had begun to scream that lightning-strike-of-hunger scream, so I was saying to him, wait just a minute let me smooth this crease, and he was shrieking a crescendo and the phone rang. While I was thinking about whether, really, we could afford new bicycles for the girls, the used ones never seem to work quite right, surely it's not such an extravagance, new bikes, but if you've been to Toys-R-Us lately you realize this is a serious issue. On the other hand, I was the fourth child and never had anything new, so I understand the dream, that lust, for something smooth and shiny and unmarked and smelling like paint and not like old garbage mildew. So I was thinking: maybe I should try to work another job, after all I am a doctor.

DOCTOR: *[Holding up her hand as if on the phone]* Hi, how are you? Yes, I'm Dr. Martin . . .

MOTHER: . . . pointing to the name tag that says "Dr. Martin" on the white coat that says doctor, doctor, doctor . . .

DOCTOR: *[Still on the phone, but now as a flashback to an earlier incident when she answered the phone]* You're having trouble breathing, Mr. Dantio? Pain in your side, a little nausea? The pills bothering you? So sorry to hear about your son. You must take care of yourself. No one can tell you for sure that you're going to die. It's a bad disease but there are always exceptions . . .

PERSON: God, hold my hand god. Where in medical school did I miss that course on conviction, so I could say, THIS IS WHAT YOU SHOULD DO, MR. DANTIO.

MOTHER: And me still folding diapers, patting them into squares warm and fresh from the dryer.

DOCTOR: *[On the phone]* I don't know, Mr. Dantio. The cancer is all over your lungs.

PERSON: Those cells are eating you, collapsing you, deflating you. Your x-ray looks like a drowned man, and each breath drives a spike of pain through your chest. Your wife sits in the corner and hates you and loves you and hates you. I see it in her eyes.

DOCTOR: *[On the phone]* I don't know when can life end . . .

[During Person's long monologue Doctor should lower her hand to indicate she is no longer on the phone.]

PERSON: Myself I would rather die, but I'm a coward, always have been. I admire your ferocity — I can't help, I can't win this battle, slay the dragon . . . , oh I want to be the hero now. I'll hold your hand, Mr. Dantio. I'll watch when you scream and the water in your lungs bubbles up pink like cotton candy from your mouth and nostrils and I'll see the terror in your eyes as you try to pull a breath and your muscles contract and your ribs stand out like a skeleton and no air comes in and your children live three thousand miles away and hate you and love you and your wife is sobbing in the corner. I'm the doctor and I'm supposed to DO SOMETHING, the other doctors say why don't you scope him, biopsy him, give him a bit of chemo, cut him, needle him, anything but don't just let him die and Mr. Dantio I'm not just letting you die, it wasn't my decision, no one asked me should he live or die. But all I can do is watch, I will do that, I will watch even the very end when the air won't come and your fingers claw against the rails on the bed *[Pause]* and you said . . .

DANTIO: No painkillers doctor, I want to see it coming.

DOCTOR: Are you sure?

PERSON: Oh, god.

DOCTOR: Do you remember when we first met, Mr. Dantio? And you complained that you itched, and it was flea bites? And you had headaches, and it was because your wife yelled at you and you yelled at her? You would call me in the middle of the night, and I would jump when the phone rang, my husband would groan and roll over in bed, one of the girls would start to cry, and the page operator said with a clothespin clipped on her nose: *[Imitating operator's nasal voice]* "Mr. Salvadore Dantio for you, Dr. Martin." And I would wake up and you would say . . .

DANTIO: Doctor, is that you doctor? Listen, I can't sleep for the itching.

PERSON: And there was nothing wrong with you and I hated you, but in the morning you would say . . .

DANTIO: I'm sorry. Sorry. Things get so bad in the middle of the night.

PERSON: . . . and what could I do but laugh, because it's true.

MOTHER: I didn't have clinic every day because I was supposed to do research and teach. I was the first woman doctor at the hospital, I was a role model, I was shiny and new and people whispered.

PERSON: So we met like lovers in the halls and in the lobbies.

DOCTOR: Really, you should try to come to your appointments, Mr. Dantio. I'll just squeeze you in today. Meet me on the second floor, but next time KEEP YOUR APPOINTMENT.

MOTHER: . . . and my friends said you'll never get ahead seeing patients in your research time like that.

DOCTOR: Mr. Dantio, there is nothing wrong with you but your wife and your kids and your boss.

MOTHER: You put your bony fingers over my hand and said . . .

DANTIO: How's a young girl like you a doctor?

MOTHER: And I laughed. You drove me crazy.

DOCTOR: I'm forty, Mr. Dantio. Forty.

PERSON: And I don't know how to live. And you finally did get something wrong with you, Salvadore. You sure did.

MOTHER: The phone is ringing and the baby is crying and I just want to finish folding the diapers so I can balance them on top of the blue and yellow receiving blankets, which is why I didn't use bleach, which I should have because there is a large brown stain on one of the diapers. How did this happen to me? I swore never a housewife, never, never, I won't fall in that black hole, not me. You grabbed my hand in that cold white room, Mr. Dantio, and you said,

DANTIO: [Sounding physically weak but firm in conviction] I'm a fighter, but only if there's a chance. All these doctors want to cut me, stick tubes in me. I don't really understand. I'm just a salesman. Now cake decorations, that's something I understand. You tell me what I should do.

DOCTOR: I can't tell you that, Mr. Dantio, Salvadore. I'm not you.

DANTIO: Honey, I need your help.

MOTHER: . . . and you made your wife, sobbing in the corner, leave the room, and you looked at me and I thought of you lying in the ICU, with tubes in your mouth and arms and lungs and penis, and nurses ripping the sheet off and turning your stiff blue body and brushing your hair and calling you sweetie, while your blank brown eyes look up at the ceiling. You, who never wanted a lady doctor, who never wanted to be called sweetie, who always wanted to do the honey-sweetie calling.

PERSON: They're adjusting that tube in your penis and your hairless testicles are flopping from side to side, and no one even bothers to draw the curtain because your eyes are like mirrors: respirator, manometer, IV pump, EKG. Your heart keeps on going blip thump, blip thump, and your lungs and your liver and your bone marrow filled with infection and your infection is so much like you that we are killing you both together.

MOTHER: And you asked me,

DANTIO: What should I do?

DOCTOR: I'm not God.

DANTIO: Well?

MOTHER: And you looked out in the hall to make sure your wife wasn't coming in, and we were running out of time, and I stroked my nine months' pregnant belly and the baby kicked.

DOCTOR: Studies show, Mr. Dantio, that sometimes, if you have this biopsy and we treat you with antibiotics, antifungals, antivirals, you might live longer.

DANTIO: Don't tell me about studies. Tell me what you would do.

DOCTOR: Studies are important, Mr. Dantio. This is the way doctors know what to do. It's scientific and more systematic than just one doctor's experience.

MOTHER: I was good at that stuff, even though women aren't supposed to be. I knew studies and talked fast, clear, and incisive and honor society. Until then I was good at being a doctor.

DANTIO: Please.

MOTHER: I felt my breath clot up somewhere in my throat. I looked at your eyes, your ferocious eyes and I said,

DOCTOR: Mr. Dantio, Salvadore, I would not do it.

PERSON: Don't do it. Don't let them, me, do it to you. No.

MOTHER: And I couldn't stop the tears. I kissed you and waddled out of the room and stood around the corner so your wife couldn't see me, and I cried right there in the middle of the hall, with my white coat split down the middle and my belly sticking out, the baby writhing like a snake making ripples in my navy-blue maternity dress with the little red bow on top. The surgeon came up to me, a young man, younger than me, so energetic and clean shaven.

SURGEON: Did you talk him into it?

MOTHER: And he ignored the tears and the belly and the baby kicking. So unprofessional.

DOCTOR: No.

SURGEON: No?!

DOCTOR: I know, as a doctor I should have said do it, but as a person I felt . . .

PERSON: No, no, no . . .

SURGEON: There is no difference between how you feel as a doctor and as a person.

MOTHER: And I saw him with his clean white coat buttoned down the front and his neat black hair. Actually, he was a friend of mine. I was looking up because he is taller.

DOCTOR: Yes, I can see that.

MOTHER: I should have been angry or distant or something, but I wasn't, it would be a lie to say I was — I was feeling . . .

PERSON: No, I'm no doctor. I never thickened and rooted and became "Doctor." Something's wrong with me, I'm a lost pregnant woman with greasy hair and a discharge in my pants because the baby's coming and I don't know what to do because they never really helped me — Plato, Aristotle, Kant, Proust, James. All I know is this man Salvadore Dantio is dying and I can't do a thing.

MOTHER: I'm still folding the diapers. I have to do a load every day to keep up, and the phone is ringing and all I could say was . . .

DOCTOR: I will be there, Mr. Dantio.

PERSON: When your pupils fix and dilate, when your jaw slackens and

droops. I'll look through your teeth into the black cavern of your body.
I'll smell the diarrhea as your bowels let loose with blood and shit.

DOCTOR: I'll stay, Mr. Dantio.

PERSON: I won't look away. They lied to me about maternity leave. They
said, well we think you don't really want to be a doctor anyway. You
must be conflicted to have a child, want to take two months off.

MOTHER: No one sent me flowers. They send flowers to all the wives of the
doctors, but no one sent me anything, not even a card, when I came
back after three weeks still bleeding. I was the only woman doctor in
the hospital. Anyway, you never wanted a woman doctor, Mr. Dantio,
Salvadore. But in the end, you looked straight into my eyes, Salvadore,
and I couldn't lie to you. Not to you.

[Pause]

I ran into your wife in the supermarket last week over the oranges,
and she saw me and began to cry, and I put my arm around her and
tried not to cry myself.

MRS. D: You know, when he died that Sunday, I tried to call you, but they
jumped on him and pounded his chest and cut it open and squeezed his
heart. He never wanted all of that.

MOTHER: . . . and she cried, and I wondered if she knew that they did it for
me, the other doctors, because they knew I didn't want him to die.
They couldn't watch him go, so they cut him up for me. They were embarrassed for me. I cared so much I made a spectacle of myself, standing in the hall crying. And when they took a piece of his lung, after he
died, they found the infection. All I could think of was . . .

PERSON: Maybe I was wrong, maybe he could have lived longer if he'd had
that biopsy. Maybe I never learned this language right, medicine. I feel
like a visitor from some other world, dressed up like a doctor, but they
can tell I'm not really one. In moments of great stress I revert to my native tongue.

MOTHER: Mrs. Dantio wiped her eyes with the back of her hand and said,

MRS. D: Is that the baby?

MOTHER: And she looked at his smooth skin, my little son, and she smiled
and touched the drool on his chin. I laughed too.

[*Pause*]

He's still crying and I pick up the phone, and someone says, Is this the lady of the house? And I don't know what to answer, so I think but I still don't know. So I hang up and reach for the baby. He's beginning to make those enunciated baby complaints. I pull up my shirt and my breasts hang out like a cow and just looking at him I feel that sweet pain contraction. The milk spurts, and gets us wet. He makes snuffling noises, he works his mouth searching for the nipple. So I help him. Wham! he latches on and pulls, and the milk is pouring out of both breasts now. I grab a diaper to hold over the other one, but it's too late and we're drenched. He and I a milk shower. I know what this means: another load of laundry.

END

QUESTIONS FOR DISCUSSION

Why is the protagonist upset?

What is the significance of her doing the laundry as she recalls her interactions with and care of Mr. Dantio? How does she feel about being both mother and doctor? How do her colleagues feel about her being both a mother and a doctor?

Did being a mother or a feeling person affect her care of Mr. Dantio?

Did she do right by Mr. Dantio? How would you have responded to Mr. Dantio's questions and requests?

What does the *Person* character mean when she says of herself: "Maybe I was wrong, maybe he [Mr. Dantio] could have lived longer if he'd had that biopsy. Maybe I never learned this language right, medicine. I feel like a visitor from some other world, dressed up like a doctor, but they can tell I'm not really one. In moments of great stress I revert to my native tongue." What does she consider to be her "native tongue" in this context?

How was the protagonist treated by her peers? Did her being a woman make a difference to them? Should it?

Is it surprising to learn that physicians can be uncertain about the decisions they make about patients? Or that they have feelings about their patients that might affect patient care or patient/physician interactions?

What does the surgeon mean by saying that there is no difference between how you feel as a physician and how you feel as a person? Do you agree?

What did you think about the way Mr. Dantio died?

Was the protagonist a good physician? Is she too emotionally involved with her patients to provide good objective care?

What do you make of the ending of the story? Of the "milk shower"?

Imelda

RICHARD SELZER

Adapted for Readers' Theater by Gregory A. Watkins

CAST

Dr. Franciscus (Dr. F)

Medical Student (Student)

Nurse

Mother

Dr. A

Imelda

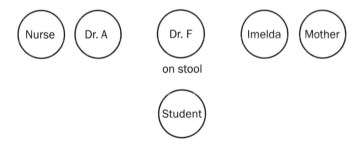

on stool

NOTES

Medical Student, Nurse, *and* Dr. A *may be played by males or females.*

Imelda *has only one word to speak in the entire story, but she appears "on stage" at several crucial points. A young teenage girl would be a good choice for this role. (However, we have used girls and women of all ages as* Imelda, *and the story remains powerful regardless of who plays the role. That is the beauty of readers' theater — the audience members use their imaginations.)*

STUDENT: I heard the other day that Hugh Franciscus had died. I knew him once. He was the Chief of Plastic Surgery when I was a medical student at Albany Medical College. Dr. Franciscus was the archetype of the professor of surgery — tall, vigorous, muscular, as precise in his technique as he was impeccable in his dress. Each day a clean lab coat monkishly starched, that sort of thing.

NURSE: I doubt he ever read books. One book only, that of the human body, took the place of all others. He never raised his eyes from it. He read it like a printed page, as though he knew that in the calligraphy there just beneath the skin were all the secrets of the world.

DR. A: Long before it became visible to anyone else, even to us on the medical staff, Franciscus could detect the first sign of granulation at the base of a wound, the first blue line of new epithelium at the periphery that would tell him a wound would heal, or the barest hint of necrosis that presaged failure. This ability gave him the appearance of a prophet.

DR. F: *[Stands] [Spoken with authority]* This skin graft will take.

DR. A: And you must believe — that it would.

[Dr. F sits.]

STUDENT: He had enemies, of course, who said he was arrogant, that he exalted activity for its own sake. Perhaps. But perhaps it was no more than the honesty of one who knows his own worth. Just look at a scalpel, after all. What a feeling of sovereignty, megalomania even, when you know it is you, and you alone, who will make certain use of it.

NURSE: It was said, too, he was a ladies' man. I don't know about that. It was all rumor. Besides, I think he had other things in mind than mere living.

DR. A: Franciscus was an avid hunter. Every fall during the season he drove upstate to hunt deer. There was a glass-front case in his office where he showed his guns. People asked, "How could he shoot a deer?" But he knew better.

STUDENT: To us medical students he was someone heroic, someone made up of several gods, viewed from a distance, and always from a lesser height. If *he* had grown accustomed to his miracles, *we* certainly had not.

DR. A: He had no close friends among us staff physicians. And there was something a little sad in that, as if once, long ago, he'd been flayed by friendship, and now the slightest breeze might hurt. Confidences resulted in dishonor. Maybe the person in whom he confided would scorn him, betray him. Even though he spent his days among those less fortunate, weaker than he was — the sick, after all — Franciscus seemed aware of a personal harshness in his environment. He reacted by keeping his own counsel, and was often remote. It gave him the appearance of being haughty.

NURSE: We nurses knew that with patients he was completely forthright. All the facts laid out, every question anticipated and answered, always with specific information. And he delivered good news and bad with the same dispassion.

STUDENT: I was a third-year student, just turned onto the wards for the first time and clerking on Surgery. Everything was terrifying — the operating room, the morgue, the emergency room, the patients, professors, even the nurses. I picked my way through the mines and booby traps of the hospital, hoping just to avoid the hemorrhage and perforation of disgrace. And the opportunity for humiliation was everywhere.

NURSE AND DR. A: We all felt that way.

STUDENT: It began on Ward Rounds.

[Dr. F stands.]

Dr. Franciscus was demonstrating a skin graft he had constructed to cover a large, fleshy defect in the leg of a merchant seaman who had injured himself in a fall. The man was from Spain, and spoke no English.

NURSE: There had been a fracture of the femur, a lot of tissue damage, and necrosis. After weeks of debridement and dressings, the wound had been made ready for grafting. When we saw him, the patient was in his fifth postoperative day.

STUDENT: What we saw was a thick web of pale blue flesh rising from the man's left thigh, which had been sutured to the open wound on the right thigh. Franciscus pressed the pedicle with his finger, and it blanched. When he let up, there was a slow return of the color.

DR. F: *[Spoken with authority]* The circulation is good. It will get better. In several weeks, I'll divide the tube of flesh at its site of origin, and tailor it to fit the defect. By then it will have grown more solid.

NURSE: The patient reached out and grabbed Dr. Franciscus by the arm. He started speaking rapidly, and pointing at his groin and hip. Dr. Franciscus stepped back at once and disengaged his arm.

DR. F: Anyone here speak Spanish? I didn't get a word of that.

STUDENT: *[Looking up, as if speaking to someone on a pedestal]* The cast is digging into him up above. The edges of the plaster are rough, and when he moves they hurt.

NURSE: Dr. Franciscus took plaster shears from the dressing cart and cut away the rough edges of the cast. The patient smiled, and said, *"gracias, gracias."*

STUDENT: But Dr. Franciscus had already moved on to the next bed.

[Dr. F sits.]

He seemed to me a man of immense strength and ability, but without affection for his patients. He didn't want to be touched by them. The only kindness he showed them was a reassurance that he would never give up, that he would make every effort. If anyone could, he would solve the problems of their flesh.

DR. F: You speak Spanish.

STUDENT: I lived in Spain for two years.

DR. F: I'm taking a surgical team to Honduras next week, to operate on the natives down there. I do it every year for three weeks, somewhere. This year, Honduras. I can arrange the time away from your duties here if you'd like to come along. You will act as interpreter. I'll show you how to use the clinical camera. What you'd see would make it worthwhile.

STUDENT: So, a week later, the envy of my classmates, I joined the mobile surgical unit — surgeons, anesthesiologists, nurses, and equipment — aboard a Military Air Transport plane. Three weeks performing plastic surgery on people who had already been selected by an advance team.

DR. A: Off to Honduras. From the plane, it seems to be made of clay — burnt umber, raw sienna, dry. It has a deadweight quality, as if the ground has no buoyancy, no air sacs a breeze might wander through.

STUDENT: I don't suppose I'll ever see it again. Nor do I especially want to.

NURSE: Our destination was Comayagua, a town in the central highlands.

The town itself is situated on the edge of one of the flatlands networked between the granite mountains. Higher up, everything is brown, with only an occasional Spanish cedar tree. Down below, patches of luxuriant tropical growth.

STUDENT: The town is a day's bus ride from the airport. It kept appearing and disappearing from view, with the convolutions of the road. The drive in was all I'd see of the countryside.

DR. A: The hospital itself is a derelict, with the smell of spoiling bananas and the accumulated odors of everyone who'd been sick there for the last hundred years.

STUDENT: Of the two, I think I preferred the frank smell of the sick.

NURSE: And, of course, there's the heat. Incendiary. It was so hot that, as we stepped from the bus, our words couldn't carry through the air. They just hung there, limp.

STUDENT: There's a courtyard in front of the hospital, and mobs of people were waiting there, squatting or lying in the meager shade. On dry days, a fine dust would sweep through the courtyard, battering the untethered goats and the gaunt, dejected men who stood there. Those men were like their country — solemn, leaden. No one looked at the sky. Every head was bent beneath a wide-brimmed straw hat.

DR. A: They are called mestizos — mixed Spanish and Indian blood. They had broad, flat, dumb museum feet. At first, the people are indistinguishable one from another, without animation. All the vitality, the hidden sexuality, was in their black hair. We came to know them by the deep lines with which each face was graven. Even so, compared to us they were masked, shut away.

STUDENT: My job was to follow Dr. Franciscus around, photograph the patients before and after surgery, interpret, and generally act as aide-de-camp. It was exhilarating. Within days I'd decided I was not just useful, but essential. Still, even though we were together all day, there were no overtures of friendship from Dr. Franciscus. He knew my place, and I knew it, too.

DR. A: We examined patients in the afternoon, the ones scheduled for the next morning's surgery.

STUDENT: I would call out a name from the doorway to the examining room. Someone in the courtyard would rise. I would usher the patient in, and nudge him to the examining table where Dr. Franciscus stood, always, I thought, on the verge of irritability. I would read the case history aloud, then wait while he carried out the examination. While I took the "before" photographs, Dr. Franciscus would dictate into a tape recorder.

DR. F: *[Dictating — can hold hand near mouth as if holding a dictating microphone]* Ulcerating basal cell carcinoma of the right orbit — six by eight centimeters — involving the right eye and extending into the floor of the orbit. Operative plan: wide excision with enucleation of the eye. Later, bone and skin grafting.

STUDENT: We were more than two weeks into our tour of duty — a few days to go — when it happened. Earlier in the day I had caught sight of her through the window of the dispensary. A thin, dark Indian girl about fourteen years old. She looked like a hand over mouth figurine — orange-brown, terra-cotta, and still attached to the unshaped clay from which she'd been carved. Her mother — short, dumpy, sun-weathered — stood behind her, wearing a broad-brimmed hat with a high crown and a shapeless dress like a cassock.

The girl had long, loose black hair, and there were tiny gold hoops in her ears. The dress she wore could have been her mother's. Far too big, it hung from her thin shoulders as if it would fall down her arms at any moment. Even with her in it, the dress was empty — something hanging on the back of a door. Her breasts made only the smallest imprint in the cloth, her hips none at all.

And all the while, she pressed to her mouth a filthy, pink, balled-up rag, as if to stanch a flow or as a buttress against pain. I knew that what she had come to show us, what we were there to see, was hidden behind that rag. As I watched, the mother handed her a hollowed gourd, from which the girl drank, lapping like a dog. She was the last patient of the day. They had been waiting for hours.

"Imelda Valdez," I called out.

[Imelda and Mother rise. Imelda holds her right hand to her mouth as if clenching a rag to it. Imelda and Mother look straight ahead over and past the audience.]

Slowly, she rose to her feet, the cloth never leaving her mouth, and followed her mother to the examining-room door. I shooed them in.

"Imelda, you sit up there on the table. Mother, you stand over there, please."

[Mother sits.]

I read from the chart. "This is a fourteen-year-old girl with a complete, unilateral, left-sided cleft lip and cleft palate. No other diseases or congenital defects. Laboratory tests, chest x-ray, negative."

[Dr. F stands.]

DR. F: Tell her to take the rag away.

STUDENT: *Quita el trapo.* The girl shrank back, pressing the cloth to her face more firmly.

DR. F: Listen, this is silly. Tell her I've got to see it. Either she behaves, or send her away.

STUDENT: *Por favor. Dame el trapo.* I asked her to give me the cloth as gently as possible. She didn't. She couldn't.

[In this next sequence, on the words "Dr. Franciscus reached up," Dr. F should reach up and straight out with his right hand as if grabbing Imelda's rag as Imelda stands in front of him, and on the word "jerk," he should pull down as if yanking the rag from her face. Imelda, on the word "jerk," should move her right arm down and her head to the right as if jerked, then fling her right arm back at her face as described. On the words "she relaxed and sat still," Imelda should drop her arm to her side.]

Just then, Dr. Franciscus reached up and, taking the hand that held the rag, pulled it away with a hard jerk. For an instant, the girl's head followed the cloth as it left her face, one arm upflung against showing her secret. Against all hope, she would hide herself. But, a moment later, she relaxed and sat still. At that point, she seemed to me like an animal that looks outward at the infinite, at death, without fear, with nothing but recognition.

DR. F: That's better.

STUDENT: Set as it was in the center of her face, the defect was utterly hideous — a nude rubbery insect that had fastened itself there. The upper lip was widely split all the way to the nose. One white tooth perched on the protruding upper jaw, projecting through the hole. Some of the bone seemed to have been gnawed away as well. Above the thing, her clear almond eyes and long black hair reflected the light. Below it, her pulse trilled visibly in her slender neck. As we looked at her, her eyes fell to her lap, where her hands lay palms upward, half open. She was a beautiful bird with a crushed beak. And tense with the expectation of more shame.

DR. F: Open your mouth.

STUDENT: *Abre* [pronounced "abray"] *la boca*, I translated, and she did. Dr. Franciscus tipped back her head, to see inside.

DR. F: The palate, too. Complete. *[Pause]* What is your name? *¿Cómo se* [pronounced "say"] *llama* [pronounced "yama"]?

IMELDA: Imelda. *[Try to say this as described in story: "the syllables leaked through the hole with a slosh and a whistle."]*

DR. F: Tomorrow, I will fix your lip. *Mañana* [pronounced "manyana"].

STUDENT: In spite of his years of experience, in spite of all the dreadful things he'd seen, he must have been awed by the sight of this girl. I could see it flit across his face for an instant. Maybe it was her small act of concealment, that he had had to force her to show it to him. Maybe it was her resistance that intensified the disfigurement. Had she brought her mouth to him willingly, without shame, she would have been no more or less than any other patient.

[Pause] He measured the defect with calipers, studied it from different angles, turning her head with a finger at her chin.

DR. F: Take her picture. Imelda, *mira aquí* [pronounced "akee"], look straight ahead.

STUDENT: Through the eye of the camera, she seemed more pitiful than ever, her humiliation more complete.

DR. F: *[Giving an order — no urgency]* Wait!

STUDENT: A strand of hair had fallen across her face and found its way to her mouth. Dr. Franciscus removed the hair and tucked it behind her ear.

DR. F: There. Go ahead.

STUDENT: I took the photo.

DR. F: Take three more, just in case.

STUDENT: I did. Imelda and her mother left.

[Imelda and Dr. F sit.]

> I turned to Dr. Franciscus. "How can it ever be put back together?" He took paper and a pen and, with a few lines, drew a remarkable likeness of her face.

DR. F: Look, this dot is A, and this one is B, this, C, and this, D; the incisions are made A to B, then C to D. CD must be equal to AB. It's all equilateral triangles.

STUDENT: Good, but then he got to X and Y, and rotation flaps, and the rest.

DR. F: Do you see?

STUDENT: It's confusing.

DR. F: It's simply a matter of dropping the upper lip into a normal position, then crossing the gap with two triangular flaps. It's geometry.

STUDENT: "Yes," I said. "Geometry." And relinquished all hope of becoming a plastic surgeon.

DR. A: The following morning we performed the surgery. I served as anesthesiologist.

STUDENT: Imelda was already under when Dr. Franciscus and I arrived from Ward Rounds. The tube emerging from her mouth was pressed against her lower lip, to be kept out of the field of surgery. A nurse was scrubbing her face, in a reddish-brown lather. Her tiny gold earrings were included in the scrub. Now and then, one of the earrings gave a brief, brave flash. The nurse washed her face for the last time and dried it. Green towels were placed over her face, to hide everything but the mouth and nose.

DR. F: *[Dr. F stands.]* Calipers.

STUDENT: He measured, locating the peak of the distorted Cupid's bow.

DR. F: Marking pen.

STUDENT: He placed the first blue dot at the apex of the bow. The nasal sills were dotted. The A flap and the B flap were outlined. On he worked, peppering the lip and nose with blue dots, making sense out of chaos, envisioning the lip that lay in that deep, essential pink. The lip only he could see. The last dot and line were placed. He was ready.

DR. F: Scalpel. *[Pause]* Okay to go ahead?

DR. A: Yes.

STUDENT: He lowered the knife to cut.

DR. A: *[Dr. A jumps up.] [This next sequence of lines should be clipped, quick, and tense.]* No! Wait! Hold it!

DR. F: What's the matter?

DR. A: Something's wrong. I'm not sure. God, she's hot as a pistol. Blood pressure is way up. Pulse one eighty. Get her temperature.

STUDENT: The nurse fumbled beneath the drapes. We waited. She retrieved the thermometer. *[Student jumps up.]* One hundred seven! No, eight!!

DR. A: She's having a reaction to the anesthesia. Malignant hyperthermia. Ice! Ice! Get lots of ice!

STUDENT: I ran out the door and grabbed the first nurse I saw. "Ice! *Hielo!* Quickly! *Hielo!*" Her expression was blank. I ran to another. "*Hielo! Hielo!* For the love of God, ice." She shrugged. "*Nada,*" she said. I ran back into the operating room. "There's no ice," I told them. Dr. Franciscus had ripped off his rubber gloves and was feeling the skin of the girl's abdomen. Above his mask were the eyes of a horse in battle.

DR. A: The EKG is wild!

DR. F: I can't get a pulse!

DR. A: What the hell . . . ?

STUDENT: Dr. Franciscus reached for the girl's groin. No femoral pulse.

DR. A: EKG flat! *[Pause]* My God. *[Pause]* She's dead.

DR. F: *[Mad — incredulous]* She can't be!

DR. A: She is.

   [All sit.]

STUDENT: *[Pause]* It was noon, four hours later, when we left the operating room. The day was so hot and humid I felt steamed open like an envelope. Imelda's mother was sitting on a bench in the courtyard. In one hand, she held the piece of cloth the girl had used to conceal her mouth. As we watched, she folded it once, neatly, and then again, smoothing it, cleaning it, as if she were stroking Imelda's head, consoling her.

DR. F: *[Dr. F stands.]* I'll do the talking here.

STUDENT: He would tell her himself, in whatever Spanish he could find.

Only if she didn't understand was I to translate. I watched him brace himself, set his shoulders. How could he tell her? What? But I knew he would tell her everything, exactly as it had happened. As much for himself as for her, he needed to explain.

Suppose she screamed, though, fell to the ground, attacked him? All that hope of love . . . gone. Even in his discomfort I knew he was teaching me. The way to do it was professionally.

Now he was standing over her. When the woman saw that he didn't speak, she lifted her eyes and saw what he held crammed in his mouth to tell her. She knew, and rose to her feet.

[Mother stands.]

DR. F: *Señora.* I am sorry.

STUDENT: All at once, he seemed shorter than he was, scarcely taller than the mother. There was a place at the crown of his head where the hair had grown thin. His lips were stones. He could hardly move them. His voice was dry, dusty.

DR. F: No one could have known. Some bad reaction to the medicine for sleeping. It poisoned her. High fever. She did not wake up.

STUDENT: The woman studied his lips, as though she were deaf. He tried, but could not control a twitch at the corner of his mouth. He raised a thumb and forefinger to press something back into his eyes.

MOTHER: *[Spoken as a statement, not a question.] Muerte.*

STUDENT: Her eyes were human, deadly.

DR. F: *Sí, muerte.*

STUDENT: At that moment, he was like someone cast, still alive, as an effigy for his own tomb. He closed his eyes, and didn't open them until he felt the touch of the woman's hand on his arm, a touch from which he did not withdraw. Then he looked and saw the grief corroding her face, breaking it down, melting the features so that her eyes, nose, mouth ran together in a distortion, like her daughter's.

For a long time they stood in silence. At last, her face cleared, the features rearranged themselves. She spoke, the words coming slowly so he could understand her.

MOTHER: I go home now. Tomorrow, my sons come for Imelda, to bring her home for burial. Do not be sad. God has decided. And I am happy that her mouth has been fixed, so she can go to Heaven that way.

[Mother and Dr. F sit.]

STUDENT: *[Pause]* The next morning, I didn't go to the wards, but stood at the gate leading from the courtyard to the road outside. Two young men in striped ponchos lifted Imelda's body, wrapped in a straw mat, onto the back of a wooden cart. A donkey waited. All at once, the woman looked up and saw me. She had taken off her hat. The heavy-hanging coil of her hair made her head seem larger, darker, noble. I pressed some money into her hand. "For flowers," I said. "A priest."

MOTHER: *Sí. Sí. [Pause]* The doctor is one of the angels. He has finished the work of God. My daughter is beautiful.

STUDENT: What? I thought to myself. The lip had not been fixed. The girl had died before Dr. Franciscus had done it.

MOTHER: Only a fine line that God will erase in time.

STUDENT: I reached into the cart and lifted a corner of the mat in which the girl had been rolled. Where the cleft had been there was now a fresh line of tiny sutures. The Cupid's bow was delicately shaped, the vermilion border aligned. The flattened nostril now had the same rounded shape as the other one. I let the mat fall over the face of the dead girl, but not before I had seen the touching place where the finest black hairs sprang from the temple.

MOTHER: *Adios. Gracias.*

STUDENT: *[Pause] [Reflectively]* There are events in a doctor's life that seem to mark the boundary between youth and age, seeing and perceiving. Like certain dreams, they illuminate a whole lifetime of past behavior. After such an event, a doctor is not the same as he was before.

It had seemed to me then the act of someone demented, or at least insanely arrogant. An attempt to reorder events. Her death had come to him out of order. It should have happened after the lip had been repaired, not before.

And he could have told her mother, no, the lip had not been fixed. But he didn't. He said nothing. It had been an act of omission, one of those strange lapses we're all subject to, which we all live to regret.

It must have been then, at that moment, that the knowledge of what he would do appeared to him. The mother's words hadn't consoled him; *[with some hint of danger]* they had hunted him down. And he hadn't done it for her; the dire necessity was his. He would not accept that Imelda had died before he could repair her lip.

People who do such things break free from society. They follow their own lonely path. They have a secret they can never reveal. I must never let on that I know.

[Narrating again] But how often I've imagined it. Ten o'clock at night. The hospital at Comayagua is all but dark. Here and there lanterns tilt and skitter up and down the corridors. One of the lamps breaks free from the others and descends the stone steps to the morgue, underground.

The room has waited all night for someone to come. No silence so deep as this place, with its cargo of newly dead. Only the slow drip of water over stone.

The door closes and clicks shut.

[Dr. F stands.]

The lock is turned. There are four tables, each with a body encased in a paper shroud. There's no mistaking her. She's the smallest.

He takes a knife from his pocket and slits open the paper shroud, the part in which the girl's head is enclosed. The wound seems to be living on long after she has died. Waves of heat emanate from it, blurring his vision. He turns and peers over his shoulder, and sees nothing but the wooden crucifix on the wall. He removes a package of instruments from his satchel, and arranges them on a tray.

DR. F: *[All Dr. F's lines in this section are spoken as if muttering to himself.]* Scalpel, scissors, forceps, needle holder. Sutures, sponges.

STUDENT: Stealthy, hunched, engaged, he begins.

DR. F: The blue dots are still there, on her mouth.

STUDENT: He raises the scalpel, pauses. A second glance into the darkness. From the wall, a small lizard watches and accepts.

DR. F: The first cut. Sluggish flow of dark blood. Wipe it away with a sponge. No new blood takes its place.

STUDENT: Again and again he cuts, connecting each of the blue dots until the whole of the zigzag slice is made, first on one side of the cleft, then on the other. Now the edges of the cleft are lined with fresh tissue. He sets down the scalpel and takes up scissors and forceps.

DR. F: Undermine the flap until each triangle is attached only at one side. Rotate each flap into its new position. They must be free enough to be swung without tension. They are. I'm ready to suture. Needle into the needle holder, then each suture precisely the same distance from the cut edge, the same distance apart. Tie the knots down until the edges are apposed. Not too tightly.

STUDENT: These are the most meticulous sutures of his life.

DR. F: Cut each thread close to the knot.

STUDENT: It goes well. The vermilion border, with its white skin roll, is exactly aligned. One more stitch, and the Cupid's bow appears, as if by magic. His face shines with moisture.

DR. F: The nostril is incised around the margin, released, and sutured into a round shape to match the other.

STUDENT: He wipes the blood from her face with gauze he's dipped in water. He folds the shroud around her once more, and returns his instruments to the satchel. In a moment, the morgue is dark, and a lone lantern ascends the stairs and is extinguished.

[Dr. F sits.]

DR. A: *[Long pause]* Six weeks after we returned from Honduras, Franciscus presented his case material in the amphitheater of the medical school. It was the highlight of the year. The hall was filled.

DR. F: *[Dr. F stands and faces stage left so he can look left at "slides" behind him and right at audience in amphitheater in front of him.]* Next slide.

STUDENT: The night before, he had arranged the slides in the order in which they would be shown. I was at the controls of the slide projector.

DR. F: This is a fifty-seven-year-old man with a severe burn contracture of the neck. You will notice the rigid webbing that has fused the chin to the presternal tissues. No motion of the head on the torso is possible. Next slide. Here he is after the excision of the scar tissue and with the head in full extension for the first time. The defect was then covered. Next slide.

STUDENT: I advanced the carriage.

DR. F: *[Droning on]* . . . with full-thickness drums of skin taken from the abdomen with the Padgett dermatome. Next slide.

[Imelda stands and looks straight out past the audience.]

STUDENT: And then, suddenly, there she was, extracted from the shadows, suspended above and beyond all of us like a resurrection. There was the oval face, the long black hair unbraided, the tiny gold hoops in her ears. And that luminous gnawed mouth. The whole of her life summed up in this photograph.

DR. A: *[Stage whisper]* What? The girl from Comayagua? The one who died on the table? What in God's name is he doing?

NURSE: It went silent in the amphitheater, all of us sitting there in the dark, waiting for Dr. Franciscus to break the silence. None of us — doctors, nurses, students — knew what was going on, but no one would, or could, speak.

STUDENT: My own pulse doubled. It was hard to breathe. Why didn't he call out for the next slide? Why didn't he save himself? Why hadn't he removed this slide from the ones to be shown? And then I knew. He had used his camera on her again. I could see the long black shadows of her hair flowing into the darker shadows of the morgue. The sudden, blinding flash. The next slide would be the one taken in the morgue. He would be exposed.

DR. A: *[Stage whisper]* I have no idea what he is doing.

STUDENT: He just stood there, for what seemed like minutes, looking up at the image of the girl. In complete silence. For me, the amphitheater had become Honduras. The courtyard littered with patients. I could see the dust in the beam of light from the projector. It was then that I knew she was his measure of perfection and pain — the one lost, the other gained. He, too, had heard the click of the camera, had seen her wince.

NURSE: Finally, Dr. Franciscus spoke.

DR. F: *[Tenderly]* Imelda.

STUDENT: At the sound of his voice, I removed the next slide from the projector and hit the advance button.

[Imelda sits.]

She was gone. I hit the button again, and in her place was the man with the orbital cancer. For a long moment, Dr. Franciscus looked up in my direction, on his face an expression that I have given up trying to interpret. Gratitude? Sorrow? It made me think of the way the girl had looked, when she understood she must hand over to him the evidence of her body.

DR. F: [*In a normal voice, as though nothing had happened*] This is a sixty-two-year-old man with a basal cell carcinoma of the temple eroding into the bony orbit . . .

NURSE: Whatever had happened, it was over.

[*Dr. F sits.*]

STUDENT: At the end of the hour, even before the lights came on, there was loud applause. I hurried to find him among the departing crowd, but couldn't.

Some weeks went by before I caught sight of him. He seemed vaguely convalescent, as though a fever had taken its toll before burning out.

He continued to teach for fifteen years, though he operated a good deal less frequently, then gave it up entirely. It was as if he had grown tired of blood, of always having to be involved with blood, of having to draw it, spill it, wipe it away, stanch it. He was a quieter, softer man, I heard, his ferocity diminished. There were no more expeditions to Honduras, or anywhere else.

Nor have I been entirely free of her. Now and then, in the years that have passed, I see that donkey-cart procession, or his face bent over hers in the morgue.

And I would like to tell him what I now know, that his unrealistic act was one of goodness, one of those small, persevering acts done, perhaps, to ward off madness. Like lighting a lamp, boiling water for tea, washing a shirt. But, of course, it's too late now.

END

QUESTIONS FOR DISCUSSION

Did Dr. Franciscus do something wrong? Did he lie? Did he desecrate Imelda's body? Why were he and the student so secretive about the repair?

Why did Dr. Franciscus repair Imelda's lip?

Contrast the reactions of the various characters to Imelda's death, especially the mother's and Dr. Franciscus's. Does cultural background play a role in their reactions?

Why was Dr. Franciscus so touched by Imelda?

What kind of man was Dr. Franciscus before meeting Imelda? After? Why the change?

Why did the medical student remove the slide at the last second? Was it a justifiable action? What secret was the medical student trying to protect about Dr. Franciscus? What would the slide have revealed to those assembled at the presentation?

Why couldn't Franciscus speak when the slide of Imelda's face first appeared on the screen? Why did Franciscus change after this slide presentation?

Who is this story about? Dr. Franciscus? The medical student? Imelda? Why is it called "Imelda"?

Is this a sad story? For which characters?

What do you take away from this story? Why is the story so powerful and captivating? Is there a lesson in it?

Old Doc Rivers

WILLIAM CARLOS WILLIAMS

Adapted for Readers' Theater by Gregory A. Watkins

CAST

Reader 1 (male): Grimley, Jerry, Milliken, Trowbridge, Brother

Reader 2 (male): Rivers (standing), Druggist, John

Reader 3 (male or female): Doctor

Reader 4 (female): Nurse, Miss Jeannette

Reader 5 (female): Woman 2, 4, 6, 9, Lady, Mary

Reader 6 (female): Woman 1, 3, 5, 7, 8, Librarian, Mrs. Shippen, Girl

Reader 7 (male): Boy, Man, Dr. Jamison, Mr. Shippen, Super

The parts each reader takes can vary as required by the number of male and female performers available. An alternate distribution of parts could be:

Reader 1 (male): Grimley, Boy, Jerry, Man, Milliken, John, Super, Brother

Reader 2 (male): Doc Rivers, Dr. Jamison, Shippen, Druggist, Trowbridge

Reader 3 (male or female): Doctor

Reader 4 (female): Nurse, Mary, Miss Jeannette

Reader 5 (female): Woman 2, 4, 6, 8, Librarian, Lady, Girl

Reader 6 (female): Woman 1, 3, 5, 7, 9, Mrs. Shippen

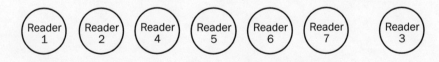

NOTES

This story is a bit more of a challenge to perform than the others because of the number of characters and the lack of a recognizable progression of events leading to a climax. "Old Doc Rivers" is a series of recollections by a physician colleague about the life of the almost legendary (in that town) Dr. Rivers. The audience hears various townspeople and physicians, including the physician-narrator, describe some of their encounters with and opinions of Rivers.

Cast members other than the one who plays Doctor *(the physician-narrator) will read a number of parts, perhaps employing various accents, styles of speaking, and standing and sitting positions to distinguish one character from another. The script is keyed for seven readers. If this configuration of readers is used, then the discussion leader should announce at the start of the performance that* Reader 2 is Dr. Rivers *when standing and other characters when seated.*

Physician impairment is a difficult but important issue. Who is responsible for reporting physicians who potentially or actually put their patients in danger because they are impaired or incompetent? What risks do colleagues and patients take in reporting such physicians? In preparation for leading a discussion of this story, the discussion leader might wish to investigate the way physician impairment is handled in his/her state by contacting the local or state medical society or by looking on those organizations' Web sites.

Readers for this script are designated R1 through R7.

R3, DOCTOR: Grimley was a young doctor *[Grimley (R1) stands.]*, a first-rate physician who began practicing in town a month or two prior to my arrival. He had it in for Rivers. My wife would sometimes say to me, "If you know Rivers is killing people, why don't you doctors get together and have his license taken away?" I would answer that I didn't know.

R1, GRIMLEY: I had a young Hungarian girl under my care with a strangulated hernia who was scared as hell of the knife. I tried my best to reduce it, but without success. I knew she was in danger, and I urged her to go to the hospital and have the operation. She refused.

R3, DOCTOR: Grimley told her that, unless she had the operation, he would no longer handle her case, that she would die.

R1, GRIMLEY: The next day she called me again. As soon as I entered the room, I could see it was all over. She had called in Rivers. He had told her he could cure her. God knows what condition he was in at the time. He'd pressed on the sac until it burst. She died the next day.

R3, DOCTOR: I met Grimley at the corner by the drug store. He wanted to have Rivers arrested.

R1, GRIMLEY: I wanted to have him prosecuted for malpractice, to put him out of the way once and for all.

R3, DOCTOR: He never did.

[Grimley sits.]

R7, BOY: *This* happened many years ago. I was sick, and my old man was worried. Finally, the druggist tipped us off. "Get Rivers," he said. "He's a dope addict, but when he's right you can't beat him. I'll call up Rivers and get him down here at the store. If he's right, I'll send him up." Later in the day, the Doc came into my room and took one look at me. "This boy's got typhoid fever," he said. Just like that — that's how he did it. And sure enough, he was right. He had the jump on the thing. The result was I had a light case and we had Rivers for years after that as our family physician.

R3, DOCTOR: This is how he practiced:

[Rivers (R2) and Jerry (R1) stand and face each other.]

R2, RIVERS: Come in, Jerry. How's the old soak?

R1, JERRY: For Christ's sake, Doc, lay off me. I'm sick.

R2, RIVERS: Who's sick? Have a drop of the old Crater. *[Note: He's offering Jerry a drink.]* Did a dog bite you?

R1, JERRY: Look at this damned neck of mine. *[Pause]* Jesus! What's the matter with you, Doc? Easy!

R2, RIVERS: Shut up, you white-livered Hibernian!

R1, JERRY: Aw, Doc, for Christ's sake. Give me a break.

R2, RIVERS: What's the matter? Did I do anything to you?

R1, JERRY: Listen, Doc, ain't you gonna put anything on it?

R2, RIVERS: On what? Keep those pants buttoned. Sit down. Grab onto these arms. And don't let go until I'm through or I'm likely to slit you in half.

R1, JERRY: Ow! Jesus, Mary, and Joseph! What'd you do to me, Doc?

R2, RIVERS: I think your throat's cut, Jerry. Here, drink this. I didn't think you were so yellow. Go lie down over there for a minute.

R1, JERRY: Lie down? What for? What do you think I am, a woman? You got any more of that liquor? *[In gratitude]* You're some man, Doc. Some man. What do I owe you?

R2, RIVERS: That's all right, Jerry. Bring it around next week.

[Rivers freezes; Jerry sits.]

R3, DOCTOR: Or like this:

[Woman 1 (R6) stands, faces Rivers.]

R6, WOMAN 1: *[Weakly]* Doctor?

R2, RIVERS· Yes, I know. Where is it? In your belly?

R6, WOMAN 1: Yes, Doctor.

R3, DOCTOR: A quick examination, slipping on a rubber glove after washing his hands at the basin in the corner of the room. The whole thing took less than six minutes.

R2, RIVERS: *[Rivers faces Woman 1.]* Get this prescription filled. Take thirty drops of it tonight, in a little water. And here, here's a note to Sister Rose. Get up to the hospital in the morning. And don't eat any breakfast.

R6, WOMAN 1: What's the matter with me?

R2, RIVERS: *[Dismissive]* Now, now. Tomorrow morning. Don't worry, Mother. It'll be all right. Good-bye.

[Rivers freezes; Woman 1 sits.]

R7, MAN: He loved to ride. Loved to sit back in the carriage, have a smoke, and ride. He was proud of his teams of horses, too. Of course, it was the teams got him where he needed to be.

R3, DOCTOR: He must have given value for value, good services for money received. He had a record of thirty years behind him, of getting there (provided you could find him), anywhere, anytime, for anybody — no distinctions. And of doing something, mostly the right thing, once he was there.

[Woman 2 (R5) stands.]

R5, WOMAN 2: My son had had diarrhea for about a week, and my husband and I were frantic.

We had already called in several doctors, and they had each prescribed medicines, none of which had any effect. We finally called in Doctor Rivers. He pulled down my son's pants, and said . . .

R2, RIVERS: Hell, what he needs is a circumcision.

R5, WOMAN 2: And he did it, there and then. He wouldn't let our son eat for a day or two (because of the operation, he said), and the diarrhea went away.

R7, MAN: He was very smart. Quite a psychologist.

[Rivers and Woman 2 sit.]

R3, DOCTOR: It occurred to me to drop in at St. Michael's Hospital, where he took many of his surgical cases. To satisfy my curiosity as to the man's scope.

R6, LIBRARIAN: May I help you?

R3, DOCTOR: I'd like to look at some of your older record books.

R6, LIBRARIAN: That would be the Registry of Cases. They cover back to 1898.

R3, DOCTOR: I chose the years 1905 and 1908 and I began to thumb through the entries, looking for Rivers's name. It was all there in that hospital register. Surgically there were the usual scrapings. Appendicitis was common. Endometritis, salpingitis, contracture of the hand, ruptured spleen, hernia. There were malignancies of the bowel, breast amputations, and here an ununited fracture of the humerus involving the insertion of a plate and marked "cured." The normal maternity cases, Cesarean sections, ruptured ectopic pregnancies, fistulas, hysterectomies, gall bladder resections, even a deviated septum. And at the far edge of the page the brief legend, "cured," followed his name as often as that of any other doctor. The same was true of the medical cases he treated.

[Dr. Jamison (R7) stands.]

R7, JAMISON: Sometimes, though, we doctors well knew, he'd have to quit an operation and have one of us finish it for him. Or he'd retire for a moment (we all knew why) and return, change his gloves, and continue. The transformation in him would be striking. From a haggard old man he would be changed "like that" into a resourceful and alert operator.

R3, DOCTOR: I asked some of the people who had worked with him their opinion of him as a doctor, starting with his nurse.

[Nurse (R4) stands.]

R4, NURSE: Dr. Jamison, an intern at the hospital, woke up one morning and found Doctor Rivers asleep on his bed, outside the covers, snoring away. And once, on a trip to Nashawan Hospital for Mental Diseases, an orderly found him leaning against a wall, in a semiconscious condition.

R3, DOCTOR: Something had gone wrong with his usual arrangements, and he was coked to the eyes.

R7, DR. JAMISON: He had an uncanny sense for diagnosis. He never floundered. He made up his mind and went to it. And he wasn't radical or eccentric in his surgical technique, but conservative and thoroughgoing throughout. He was cool and painstaking — so long as he had the drug in him. And he wasn't an exhibitionist in any sense of the word.

[Jamison sits. Rivers (R2), Woman 3 (R6), and Milliken (R1) stand.]

R6, WOMAN 3: My husband had a case of appendicitis, and we called in Doc Rivers. The only room big enough to handle him in was the parlor, so we rigged up a table there. Doc told my husband to climb up on the table, and he did.

R4, NURSE: Her husband, Mr. Milliken, was quite a drinker. Doctor Rivers told his assistant to give him some ether. It didn't take long — not more than twenty minutes — to see that ether wouldn't touch this fellow any way you gave it to him. He was big as a horse, and seemed as strong, too. Doctor Rivers started anyway.

R6, WOMAN 3: My husband asked Doc to hold on a minute, so Doc told his assistant to go ahead and use the chloroform.

R4, NURSE: He administered it himself, enough to put down an army. To no effect. Every time the Doctor touched Milliken with a scalpel, the man's knees flew up to his chest. Finally, we had to hold him down, all of us, while the Doctor performed the operation. It was all we could do to keep him still. It's a wonder the operation went as well as it did.

R6, WOMAN 3: I was with my husband, a month or so later, when we ran into the Doc in front of the firehouse.

R2, RIVERS: You look well enough, Milliken. Did you feel anything during the operation?

RI, MILLIKEN: Did I feel anything? My God! Every bit of it. Every bit of it.

R6, WOMAN 3: But he was well.

[Rivers, Woman 3, and Milliken sit.]

R3, DOCTOR: And there was Frankel, a friend of mine. I was called in to assist, and when I arrived, they had already rigged up the kitchen as an operating room. There were sterile dressings, instruments boiling on the gas stove, and everything was in good order.

R4, NURSE: The Doctor called Mr. Frankel into the kitchen.

R3, DOCTOR: I was stunned. Frankel had been in bed in the front of the house. He came into the kitchen in bare feet and an old-fashioned nightgown, holding his painful belly with both hands.

R4, NURSE: Doctor Rivers told Mr. Frankel to climb up on the table.

R3, DOCTOR: Frankel was simply too sick for that. Still, he got up on the table, where we put another sheet over him and started the anesthetic. Rivers asked Frankel's wife if she had any whiskey, and she brought him a bottle. He poured himself nearly a tumblerful, filled the glass with water from the sink, and began to drink.

R4, NURSE: He offered us a drink, but we declined.

R3, DOCTOR: He finished his drink, and after that things went pretty much according to surgical practice. He made the incision. He took one look and shrugged his shoulders. It was a ruptured appendix. He shoved in a drain and let it go at that, the right thing to do. But Frankel died the next day. People talked:

[Man (R7) stands.]

R7, MAN: Another decent citizen done to death by that dope fiend.

R3, DOCTOR: It was hard not to agree. And yet . . .

[Nurse and Man sit.]

R5, LADY: *[Elegantly]* He played the violin excellently. He would often join me for an evening, playing duets at the church.

R3, DOCTOR: And the Shippen girl.

R7, MR. SHIPPEN: My daughter, Virginia, was five, and had just had scarlet fever. There was some kind of complication with her kidneys. Doc came in day and night. He did everything that could be done to save her. Still, she didn't come around. She stayed unconscious, and her kidneys weren't working. Doc finally gave up. He told us she'd be dead by morning. But my wife wasn't ready to give up.

R6, MRS. SHIPPEN: I asked him if I could try putting flaxseed poultices over Virginia's kidneys. He said it would be all right.

R3, DOCTOR: It worked. The next day, the child's kidneys started to function — slowly; muddy stuff at first, but she was conscious and her fever had dropped. Rivers was delighted. He praised Mrs. Shippen, and told her she had taught him something. Virginia lived another thirty years.
[Rivers (R2) and Mary (R5) stand.]

R2, RIVERS: *[Rough throughout this exchange]* Well, Mary, what is it?

R5, MARY: I have a pain in my side, doctor.

R2, RIVERS: How long you had it, Mary?

R5, MARY: Today, doctor. It's the first time.

R2, RIVERS: Just today. That's all?

R5, MARY: Yes, doctor.

R2, RIVERS: Get up on the table and pull up your dress. Throw that sheet over you. Come on, come on. Up with you. Come on now, Mary. Pull up your knees.

R5, MARY: *[Hurts]* Oh!
[Rivers and Mary sit.]

R3, DOCTOR: He could be cruel and crude. And, like all who are so, he could be sentimentally tender also, and painstaking without measure.

R6, GIRL: My foster parents would never have anyone else. For months I went to him, two or three times a week. He was always gentle and patient. I had a sinus condition, very difficult to manage. Little by little, he brought me along, until I was well. He charged us next to nothing for his services. I admire him. I always will.

R3, DOCTOR: That, not money, was his reward.

R2, DRUGGIST: He came in my drugstore one day. There was a little fellow there, had a big abscess on his neck. Family hadn't been able to find

Doc in his office, so the boy had followed him to the store. "Come here," Doc says, "let's see." And with that he takes a scalpel out of his vest pocket and makes a swipe at the thing. Boy was too quick for him, though. Jerked back and the knife caught him low. He turned and ran, bleeding and yelling, out the door. Doc chuckled a bit, and went on about his business.

R4, MISS JEANNETTE: He used to visit my father, Mr. Jeannette, a lot. Not as a doctor, but as a friend.

R3, DOCTOR: The Jeannette mansion, two miles north of town along the ridge, was one of Rivers's favorite places. Mr. Jeannette, like most of the other French who had settled in that area, kept principally to his manor.

R1, TROWBRIDGE: Jeannette was Alsatian. Went back to France later, and someone else lives there now.

R3, DOCTOR: And that's how Doc got on the dope?

R1, TROWBRIDGE: Oh, Jeannette was a high liver. He built himself a greenhouse in the back of his mansion and put all kinds of plants in it. He must have spent hundreds and hundreds of dollars on it.

R4, MISS JEANNETTE: Father and Doctor Rivers would sit in the greenhouse and play cards with friends. They would talk and laugh, enjoy a cigar. Especially in winter. They would sit in the heat, sipping wine, with the snow piled all around.

R1, TROWBRIDGE: If Jeannette was a high liver, Rivers was no laggard before any lead Jeannette might propose. Still, I don't believe Jeannette doped. No, I think Rivers went there looking for safety, for haven from the crude environment of those days. The mansion was foreign, incongruous, and delightfully aloof.

R4, MISS JEANNETTE: Doctor Rivers always seemed so gay during his visits. So relaxed. Out of the reach of patients.

[Pause]

R3, DOCTOR: There were times, too, when he didn't hit the dope for months at a stretch. Then he'd get to taking it again. Finally, he'd feel himself slipping, and he'd head off, overnight sometimes, leaving his practice, for the woods.

R2, JOHN: He loved to hunt. Hunt the deer. He'd bring them home and give cuts of venison to all his friends. But that ended pretty badly. One day, after his eyes had got bad from all the abuse and illness, he accidentally shot his best friend, a guide he always followed, shot him through the temples as dead as a doornail.

R3, DOCTOR: He made amends to the family, though, as well as he could. Gave them everything that was asked of him, to the last penny.

R5, WOMAN 4: He made a hobby one time of catching rattlesnakes, which abound in the mountains. He enjoyed the sport and the danger, apparently, while there was a scientific twist to it in that the venom they collected was used for laboratory work in the city.

R7, BOY: *[Awed]* He was a great hunter. I remember one time he was telling my father how he was bitten by a rattler, on the arm. Being a doctor, he knew what he was up against. He asked his guide to take his knife and cut the place out, but the guide didn't have the nerve. So Doc took his own hunting knife in the other hand and sliced it wide open and sucked the blood out of it. I suppose he took a shot of dope first, to steady himself. He rolled up his sleeve and showed us the scar, right down the middle of his arm.

R4, NURSE: I came into the office one evening to help out as his nurse while he was in with Charlie Hansel. There were several people in the waiting room, and we all heard Doctor Rivers tell Charlie to put on the gloves — boxing gloves. He always had a couple of pairs lying around the place somewhere. Charlie told me later that he'd actually had to hit Doctor Rivers, lightly, to get him to stop. Charlie was a fine young man, you see, in much better condition than Doctor Rivers.

R3, DOCTOR: There were times when even his brother couldn't do anything with him. He'd go completely mad. He put in several sessions at the State Insane Asylum, six months and more, on at least two occasions. *[Rivers (R2) and Super (R7) stand.]*

R2, RIVERS: Well? What do you think superintendent? Can I go out to work again?

R7, SUPER: You're as good a doctor as I am, Rivers. If you think you can make it, go ahead.

[Rivers and Super sit.]

R3, DOCTOR: And back he'd turn again to the old grind.

R4, NURSE: One winter he got so low with typhoid fever it looked as if, this time, things might be over. Everyone insisted he have a nurse, but he refused. And nobody, no other doctor, wanted him as a patient, either. He was completely gone with dope and the disease. Finally, he gave in and asked for a girl he had known at Blockley Hospital, a nurse he had once seen there and admired.

R3, DOCTOR: She took on the case. As soon as he was able to be up and around again, he married her. They went to Europe for a honeymoon. No doubt, she loved him.

R6, WOMAN 5: Yes, I can remember his wife. When she first came out she was a pretty little thing, just like anybody else. But I can still see her the day she came into my store, knocking against the counters, first on one side, then the other. She was covered with diamonds — on her hands, on her neck — but she didn't seem to know where she was going. Her face seemed as small as the palm of my hand.

R3, DOCTOR: A great many of his more respectable friends left him. They'd still call him — if he was right — but he was very much distrusted.

R4, NURSE: He'd sit at the table writing a prescription and you could see his head fall down lower and lower. He'd fall asleep right there, right in front of your eyes. We would shake him every once in a while, and finally he would just get up and go out.

RI, BROTHER: When he started to hit the dope, I, as his brother, tried to get him in a hospital in the city. I knew if I could get him in the proper atmosphere I could save him. He was just too foxy, though. He liked it out there, his friends, the life, whatever it was. I couldn't move him.

R4, NURSE: One of the main things that got the other doctors down on him was his habit of going off, just disappearing sometimes. He liked to go fishing, and he was a crack shot. He'd have important cases, but that didn't make any difference. All patients could do was find another doctor.

R7, BOY: *[Still awed]* One summer, my old man had gone off on a trip somewhere and sent me to the only boarding house in town. He'd left me alone in the house the year before, and was none too pleased with some of the things I did. Doc—I don't know how he did it—got me out of there, had me come stay with him. I think he insisted I was sick, that I needed treatment, and that he needed me at his house so he could keep an eye on me.

R3, DOCTOR: Sunday mornings were the times. It was a regular show. Most of his patients were poor, and they could only come on Sundays. They'd be sitting all over the place, out in the hall, up the stairs, on the porch, anywhere they could park themselves.

R7, BOY: If it was somebody that didn't know me, he'd say I was a young doctor. I was just seventeen then. He'd give me a white coat and tell me to come on. Jesus! I thought he was great. And I'll tell you, in all those four months I never saw any of the butcheries they'd talk about. Everything he did was right. I suppose I'd think different now, but then I thought he was a wonder.

R4, NURSE: He never kept any track of money. There wasn't a book around the place. Any money he got he just shoved in his pocket. Of course, he never paid for anything, either.

R7, BOY: Clever? Boy, the Doc was there! He'd go over to his desk and you'd see him fumbling around with some instruments and right in front of you he'd give himself a shot. Unless you were wise, you wouldn't even see him do it. He was foxy, too. He'd stall for a few minutes to give it time to take effect. That was when he had anything important to do. He'd wait a few minutes, and then he'd come out steely-eyed and as steady as the best of them.

R5, WOMAN 6: His wife didn't handle it nearly as well. It made her crazy. She didn't know how to control it.

R7, BOY: I can remember one night while I was living there, he waked me up at two o'clock in the morning. It was summer, one of those hot, muggy nights. I'd been operated on too, the day before. He'd taken out my tonsils or something, and I was feeling rotten. I had to go out with him just the same. We got the old buggy and started out. We went down in the meadows — at 2 A.M., mind you — down to Mooney's saloon. He went in and left me there. Anyway, I sat there slapping mosquitoes. Mooney came out after a while and told me Doc was asleep and they didn't want to wake him. I, like a kid, said all right and just sat there. He left me in that buggy 'til 5 A.M. Jesus!

R5, WOMAN 6: Then the two of them show up at my husband's butcher shop, stamping and banging 'til my husband went down and fetched them some lamb chops out of the icebox.

R7, BOY: We went home and he cooked them up in the kitchen. He was a wonderful cook. He could make a piece of meat taste like nothing in the world.

R2, JOHN: He also spent some time with a woman who kept a regular hang-out for him. It might have been a common joint, I don't know, but that isn't the way I heard it. It was certainly in an isolated location, though. One of the old houses, like the mansions on the hill only smaller — a farmhouse likely. She was a descendant of the original builders.

R6, WOMAN 7: Hello, Jimmy. How are you? Come in, and bring your cigar with you.

R2, JOHN: That's the way it began. That's the way it always began. He would just be starting a stogie.

R6, WOMAN 7: How's the boy?

R2, JOHN: The house is still there, in much the same condition. The Doc practically lived there.

R3, DOCTOR: What was the attraction? Just one thing. Something else to take him out of it. She was a good drinker. She gave him a rest. She had also put quite a bit away. The increase in land valuations had grown enormous, and she had become wealthy selling off sections of the original farm to Polacks and promoters. She was one of those who, hearing of cities and seeing trains passing right before their eyes day and night, remain isolated — unusually childish. Hot and eccentric. Rivers would find an abandoned corner like that to crawl into.

R2, JOHN: The drink would have been enough to attract him, but Doc's lady friend, she was a woman. Maybe he never thought much of that, but she was. Plenty of woman. And she could put up a hell of a fight if she wanted to. She didn't give a good God damn for the whole blankin' world — if you could believe her when she was drunk.

R3, DOCTOR: I saw her just once, many years later, when she was completely abandoned. It was the night we had her up at the police station for running through the gates at the railroad crossing. There were five in the car. I was the police physician at the time, and they wanted me to determine whether she was drunk.

[Woman 8 (R6) stands.]

R6, WOMAN 8: *[Drunk]* Have you a sister? Have you a brother? Then tell me I'm drunk. Look at me.

R3, DOCTOR: Then she went off into an unrepeatable string of profanity.

R6, WOMAN 8: And that's what I think of you. I said it. You heard me.

[Woman 8 sits.]

R4, NURSE: As far as I know, he took all the ordinary hypnotics — morphine, heroin, and cocaine also. What dose he ever got up to, it's hard to say. I've seen three grains of morphine do no more than make a woman, lying in a maternity ward, normally quiet.

R1, TROWBRIDGE: Of course, it finally got him. He began to slip badly in the latter years, to make pitiful blunders. But this final phase was marked by that curious idolatry that sometimes attracts people to a man by the very danger of his name. They seemed to recreate him in their minds, the beloved scapegoat of their own aberrant desires — and believed that he alone could cure them. He became a legend, and indulged himself the more.

R3, DOCTOR: But he did do awful things. It's said he made the remark that all a woman needed was half her organs. The others were just a surgeon's opportunity. Half the girls of Creston were without half of theirs, through *his* offices, if you could believe his story.

R5, WOMAN 9: I didn't know him very well, but we called him in anyway. When he arrived, he asked me if I had a spare room with a bed in it. I said "yes," and he went in and stayed. I was terrified. I called everyone I could think of, and no one would have anything to do with him. At five in the afternoon his driver showed up, and away they went. I've heard his driver always knew when to show up, to the minute. Knew exactly when the dope would wear off.

R3, DOCTOR: How did he get away with it? It's a little inherent in medicine itself — mystery, cures, charms of all sorts — and he knew and practiced this black art. Toward the end of his life he had a crooked eye, and was thought to be somewhat touched.

R7, BOY: There was this lady once, and Doc managed to put her under with hypnosis. I think he was surprised it worked. But he couldn't bring her around again when he was through with the experiment. I think he got scared, and he called me to come help him get her out of his office. We finally woke her up, but it took quite an effort.

R3, DOCTOR: Some felt sorry for him. Most, though, feared him. They couldn't even attack him when they knew he had really killed someone.

R4, NURSE: He cured the sick.

R3, DOCTOR: A cure for disease? He knew what that amounted to. For of what shall one be cured? Work, in his case, through sheer intuitive ability, flooded him under. Drugs righted him. Frightened, under stress, the heart beats faster, the blood is driven to the extremities of the nerves, floods the centers of action and makes us burn. That's what he wanted, must have wanted. But the reaction from such a state must have its tonics, too. That awful fever of overwork we feel especially in the United States, he had it. A trembling in the arms and thighs, a tightness of the neck and in the head above the eyes — fast breath, vague pains in the muscles and in the feet. Followed by an orgasm, crashing the job through, putting it over in a fever heat. Then the feeling of looseness after. Not pleasant, but there it is. Then cigarettes, a shot of gin, and that's all there is to it.

R4, NURSE: When a street laborer was clipped once by a trolley car, his arm was almost severed at the shoulder. Doctor Rivers was the first one there. Such cases were his particular delight. With one look, he took in the situation as usual, made up his mind, and remarking that the arm could be of no further use to the man, amputated it there and then with a pair of bandage scissors.

R3, DOCTOR: People sought him out. They'd wait months for him. Finally, though, he did give up maternity cases toward the end. When everyone else failed, they believed he'd see them through — a powerful fetish. He would save them.

R6, GIRL: My father had always had him. He fell and broke his arm, so we called Doctor Rivers in. He came, and doped himself up right in front of us. He didn't even bother to hide it.

R3, DOCTOR: That finished it.

R6, GIRL: It was the look in his eyes. "He's crazy," my father said, "Take him away. I don't want him fooling around with me. I'll get another doctor."

R2, JOHN: He bought a good-sized lot on the square before the Municipal Building, in the center of town. Built a fine house, with a big garden and double garage, where he kept two cars always ready for service. And he continued to practice for several years, while his wife bred dogs — Blue Poms, I think — and he would take them out in the car with him on his calls, holding them in his lap. In those days, he himself never sat at the wheel.

END

QUESTIONS FOR DISCUSSION

What is your assessment of Doc Rivers? Give examples to support your view.

What do you think of the way Rivers dealt with his patients? Did he provide good medical care? What was wrong with the way he dealt with patients? Give examples.

Why did the townspeople hesitate to act on Doc Rivers's behavior? Why did the physicians of the town hesitate to act on Rivers's behavior? Do the reasons apply today?

Rivers was a substance abuser and had a lifestyle some might not approve of. Should a physician's private life matter to patients?

Do patients have realistic expectations of physicians?

Who polices physicians for substance abuse and other problems in your state? Does that organization do a good job? How should physicians be policed for these problems? (The goal of this set of questions is not to encourage the audience to bash physicians but rather to encourage discussion of the best ways to contain or manage a serious problem.)

Do you know any physicians like Doc Rivers?

PART III. ETHICAL AND SOCIAL ISSUES

⊙ ⊙ ⊙ ⊙ ⊙

Follow Your Heart

RICHARD SELZER

Adapted for Readers' Theater by Ann Bean

CAST

Doctor

Narrator

Hannah Owen (Hannah)

Ivy Lou

Inez Pope

Henry Pope (Henry)

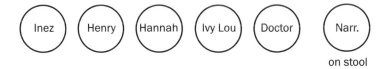

on stool

NOTES

Doctor *and* Inez Pope *are small parts. If desired, the person reading* Henry *could also read* Doctor *and the person reading* Ivy Lou *could also read* Inez Pope. *If readers do double up on parts, then they should stand for* Doctor *and for* Inez Pope *and sit for* Henry *and* Ivy Lou. Ivy Lou *can have a "country" accent.*

DOCTOR: *[Standing]* Brain dead. There is no chance that he will wake up. Ever. Look at the EEG. It's nothing but a flat line, Mrs. Owen. No blips. It's three weeks since your husband was shot in the head. The only thing keeping him alive is the respirator. I'm asking you to let us put an end to it, unplug the machinery and let him go.

NARRATOR: Hannah stared at the doctor. Let him go where, she thought. She waited for the walls of the solarium to burst.

DOCTOR: But before we do that, we would like your permission to harvest Sam's organs for transplantation.

HANNAH: Harvest? Like gathering wheat?

DOCTOR: Yes, that's what we call it when we take the organs. It's for a good cause, Hannah. In a way, your husband will live on. He will not really have died.

HANNAH: *[Staring blankly]* Dead is dead.

NARRATOR: A week later, Hannah received a letter from the doctor.

DOCTOR: *[Reading]* Dear Mrs. Owen, You will be pleased and comforted to know that because of your generosity and the miracle of modern science, seven people right here in the state of Texas are living and well, with all of their faculties restored to them. Your husband's liver has gone to a lady in McAlpine; the right kidney is functioning in Dallas; the left kidney was placed in a teenage girl in Galveston; the heart was given to a man just your husband's age in a little town near the Arkansas border; the lungs are in Fort Worth; and the corneas were used on two people right here in Houston. *[Doctor sits.]*

NARRATOR: Hannah folded the letter, put it back in its envelope and then into the bottom drawer of the desk. That was three years ago. She knew what had become of the rest of Sam. She had buried him and that was that. "Dead is dead," she had said to the doctor, but lately she wasn't so sure. Hannah had begun to have doubts. Incidents occurred, like the time, months ago, when she had gone to the butcher's. Just ahead of her at the counter, a woman had ordered a chicken. "I want it in parts," she heard the woman say. Hannah had watched as the butcher cleaved the carcass through the middle of the breast, hacked off its thighs, legs, and wings, and scooped out the entrails. The heart, gizzard, neck, and liver he put in a small plastic bag. "You can keep the feet," said the woman. Hannah turned and left just as the butcher said, "What'll it be?" After that, she stopped going to the cemetery to visit Sam's grave.

Hannah's cousin Ivy Lou, who was also her best friend, was shocked at Hannah's behavior. Ivy Lou had been born again four years ago.

IVY LOU: It's just not Christian, Hannah! What could you be thinking?

HANNAH: It isn't even Sam in that cemetery, not by a long shot. It's just parts. The parts that nobody needed. The rest of him is scattered all over Texas and very much alive. And I don't know where that leaves me. I'm thirty-three years old and a widow. If Sam were *all* dead, then maybe I could get on with my life. But this! Maybe it's a matter of percentage. If more than fifty percent of your husband is dead, then you're truly a widow.

IVY LOU: Oh, Hannah, that's a terrible thing to say. I think you ought to talk to someone about this — maybe one of Sam's doctors. This must happen to other people. Just go see someone. Ask them what they think this is all about.

HANNAH: Think! Doctors don't think, they just do! And they cover it all up with words like "harvest" and "transplantation." Why don't they say what they're really doing — "dismemberment," "evisceration."

IVY LOU: Hannah, you've got to stop this. You're driving yourself crazy and you're scaring me.

HANNAH: They make you think that you're doing the best thing, the only noble thing, and as soon as you say, "yes," they're gone.

IVY LOU: Hannah, it wasn't really like that and you know it. You told me you thought Sam would've wanted it that way.

HANNAH: And Sam . . . lately I've started to resent Sam. Here I am living in a sort of limbo and Sam's participating in seven different lives. It's not fair, Ivy Lou.

NARRATOR: Lately, Ivy Lou had taken to bringing her lunch over to eat at Hannah's. One day when she got there, she found Hannah standing at the kitchen window, staring into the backyard. Over the radio came the high-pitched monotone of a local preacher. The subject was the Resurrection of the Flesh: *[In a preaching tone]* "And it says right here in First Corinthians, chapter 15, 'For the trumpet will sound and the dead will be raised imperishable.'"

HANNAH: Turn that damn fool off!

IVY LOU: For goodness sake! What's got into you?

HANNAH: There is no such thing as the resurrection of the flesh. Just tell me at what stage of life we are supposed to be on the Day of Resurrection, so-called? Do we look as we did when we were babies? Or as we are when we die? Old and wasted? And tell me this: What about Samuel Owen on your Resurrection Day? Here he is scattered all over Texas, breathing in Fort Worth, urinating in Dallas *and* Galveston, digesting, or whatever it is the liver does, in McAlpine. Are they going to put him back together again when the Resurrection Day comes, or is it to the recipients belong the spoils? Tell me that.

IVY LOU: Well, I don't have the least idea 'bout any of that, but I do know that you are committing the sin of blasphemy! Hannah, I'm real worried about you. Don't you believe in God anymore?

HANNAH: *[Hannah slowly shakes her head and stares as she says . . .]* About God, I have only the merest inkling. That's all anyone can have.

IVY LOU: Hannah Owen, it's been three years now. You've got to accept that Sam is gone and get on with your life.

HANNAH: I know, Ivy Lou, I know. And I think I know how I can do that.

IVY LOU: Well, it's about time. I've been so worried about you.

HANNAH: I dreamed about Sam last night. I saw two men lying on narrow tables next to each other. One of them was Samuel and I couldn't tell who the other man was. The men's chests were opened, the two halves raised like cellar doors.

IVY LOU: Oh, my Lord!

HANNAH: Listen to me, Ivy Lou, please. A surgeon was there, dressed in those blue scrubs that they wear. He reached into Samuel's chest and lifted his heart out. When he held it up like a prize, it glowed. Then the surgeon turned and lowered the heart into the chest of the other man. The man immediately sat up, put on his shirt, and walked away. Then I woke up. I felt as if a weight had been lifted from me, and in that instant, I knew what I had to do. I have to find the man who is carrying Samuel's heart.

IVY LOU: What!?!

HANNAH: I know, Ivy Lou, it seemed quite mad to me at first. I asked myself, why would I do such a thing? What good would it do? The more I thought about it, the more I felt like someone whose husband has

been declared missing in action. What would I do? Why, I'd do everything I could to find him — dead or alive — until I knew one way or the
other.

IVY LOU: But, Hannah, it's not the same thing. You know that Sam really
is dead.

HANNAH: But he's not, Ivy Lou. He's alive in seven ways. I thought about
all seven of the transplantations. The liver and the lungs are hidden
away, inaccessible. And the corneas don't seem right. But the heart can
be listened to. A heart can be felt. That's what the dream meant, Ivy
Lou. I have to follow the heart.

IVY LOU: Hannah, it's . . . it's . . . sacrilegious. Like some pilgrim looking
for a shrine!

HANNAH: No Ivy Lou, it doesn't have anything to do with religion.

IVY LOU: Then what? Do you think this man will have some words of wonder for you? Even if you find him, he'd probably call the police.

HANNAH: Ivy Lou, listen to me. It doesn't have anything to do with advice
or religion. It has to do with letting go. If I can hear Sam's heart beating in this man's chest, then I can let go of Sam. *My* wound will be
healed.

IVY LOU: Hannah, I don't understand this and I don't like it at all.

HANNAH: Please try, Ivy Lou, because I need your help.

IVY LOU: My help? Whatever for?

HANNAH: I need to get ahold of Sam's medical file. Now I know that I have
a right to see it, as Sam's wife, but the hospital would remove the names
of the organ recipients first. They don't give those to the donor's family. However, as an insurance agent, I could view the *entire* file, and
that's where I need your help.

IVY LOU: Oh, no. I know what you're getting at.

HANNAH: If you could get me some letterhead stationery from your office
at Aetna Insurance Company I could call the hospital, then follow it up
with an official-looking letter.

IVY LOU: I don't like it one bit. I just don't see what you could possibly hope
to get out of this. Why, Hannah? Just tell me why?

HANNAH: [*As if wondering herself*] I don't know why.

IVY LOU: Hannah, you're going to get burned. Besides, it's not only sick, it's in the grossest ill taste!

NARRATOR: But in the end, Ivy Lou gave in. The next week at the hospital, the record librarian welcomed Hannah with a smile and showed her to a cubicle where the chart was waiting for her. Within minutes, Hannah had found the information she sought.

HANNAH: [Reading] Pope, Henry. Next of Kin: Mrs. Inez Pope. Children: None. Address: 8 Orchard Road, Avery, Texas. Diagnosis: Cardiomyopathy, viral. Surgery: Heart transplant.

NARRATOR: Hannah read on and found out that Mr. Pope's prognosis had been hopeless and he had been given an estimated life expectancy of a few months "at most." Hannah came to the details of the operation but she did not read them. She had found what she had come for. As she turned the file back in, the librarian said, "That didn't take long." Hannah replied . . .

HANNAH: No, I'm quick.

NARRATOR: Hannah looked for Avery, Texas, on the map with the help of Ivy Lou, her reluctant accomplice.

IVY LOU: There it is. Way up almost into Arkansas.

HANNAH: How far away is that?

IVY LOU: Maybe a couple of hundred miles, but Hannah, I'm telling you — don't.

NARRATOR: That night, Hannah sat at her kitchen table with a pen and a blank sheet of paper.

HANNAH: [Reading — as if considering] Dear Mr. Pope . . .

NARRATOR: She thought there was something absurd about using "Mr." considering that she had been married for seven years to a significant part of the man. But she would let it stand. The situation called for tact, diplomacy. There would be plenty of time for "Dear Henry," if and when. She picked up the pen and continued . . .

HANNAH: Dear Mr. Pope, My name is Hannah Owen. Could the name mean anything to you? Doubtless not, considering the decorum with which these things are done. I am the wife (some say widow) of Samuel

Owen, the man whose heart is even now beating in your chest. Perhaps you will forgive a woman's curiosity? I am writing to ask how you are since the operation. It is my dearest wish that the heart is doing as good a job for you as it did for Sam and for me, too. Do let me hear from you, please. Yours truly, Hannah Owen.

NARRATOR: It was two weeks before she saw the envelope in her mailbox. It was neatly addressed, in black ink, and it was postmarked Avery, Texas. It shook in Hannah's hand.

INEZ POPE: Dear Mrs. Owen, It was very kind of you to write asking after my husband's health. He is not much of a letter writer and has asked me to tell you that he is stronger and healthier than he has been in years. He says he is the luckiest man on earth. By the way, how ever did you get hold of our name and address? I thought such information might be protected, but I guess not. Thank you for your interest. Sincerely, Mrs. Inez Pope.

HANNAH: Dear Mr. Pope, I don't know any other way to say it than to just take a deep breath and come right out with it. What I am going to ask will seem at first insane. But I assure you I am no maniac. I want to come and listen to your heart for the space of one hour when it is convenient for you. While I know this request will seem strange to you, I pray that you will say yes. You have no idea how important it is to me. Yours truly, Hannah Owen.

INEZ POPE: Dear Mrs. Owen, My husband and I have tried to understand your position. But we feel that it would not be at all wise for you to come here. Not that we aren't grateful, but you have to admit it is a little on the bizarre side. So this is good-bye. Sincerely, Mrs. Henry Pope. P.S. We have consulted with our doctor who says it is a terrible idea and perhaps you should get some professional attention to get over it. No offense meant.

HANNAH: Dear *Mr.* Pope, Your wife does not wish to let me come. I can understand her hesitation. The awkwardness and all. And maybe it is only human nature to be suspicious. Perhaps I have ulterior motives? I assure you, Mr. Pope, that I do not. As for my interest in you personally, it is limited to you as the carrier of something I used to possess and which I would like to see again. Or rather, *hear* again. For that is all I want to do — to listen to your heart for the space of one hour. Your doctor doesn't think it is a good idea? Mr. Pope, the doctors don't think. If they had thought, perhaps they might have foreseen the predicament into which the "miracle of modern science" has placed me. No, speak to me not of doctors. They haven't the least idea about the human heart, except how to move it from place to place. Yours truly, Hannah Owen.

HENRY: Dear Mrs. Owen, I am very sorry. But the answer is still no. And that is final. Ever since I got your first letter, I've been feeling awful. Like an ingrate or something. But I know in my heart it wouldn't be a good thing for you either. Sincerely, Henry Pope.

HANNAH: Dear Mr. Pope, The circumstances of my husband's death were violent and shocking. In case you do not know, he was shot in the head by a bandit on the highway where he had stopped to help an old lady with a flat tire. I was there. After three weeks on life support, they came and told me it was no use, and could they disconnect the respirator? But just before they do that, could they take parts of his body ("harvest" is the word they used) to transplant to other people? I said yes, and so they took his liver, lungs, heart, corneas, and kidneys. There are seven of you out there. You, Mr. Pope, got the heart, or more exactly, *my* heart, as under the law, I had become the owner of my husband's entire body at the time he became "brain dead." Don't worry, I don't want it back. But I do ask you to let me come to Avery for one hour to listen to your heart. It is such a small thing, really, to ask in return for the donation of a human heart. Just to listen. The reasons are private, and anyway, even if I wanted to tell you why, I don't know if I could put it into words. If you see fit to let me come, I will never bother you again and you will have repaid me in full. Do please let me know when I can come. Yours truly, Hannah Owen. P.S. Of course your wife can be in the room all the time. Although frankly, I would prefer otherwise.

HENRY: Dear Mrs. Owen, You said there were seven of us recipients. Why me? Or do you plan a statewide reunion with all your husband's organs? And the answer is NO! Please do not keep writing as it is annoying to say the least, and it is making my wife nervous. Sincerely, Henry Pope.

HANNAH: Dear Mr. Pope, You ask "Why you?" And you are right to ask. It is because you have the heart. The others — the liver, lungs, kidneys — are hidden away. But the heart . . . a heart can be felt. It can be listened to. A heart is reachable. That's why you. Yours truly, Hannah Owen.

NARRATOR: When there had been no reply for two weeks, Hannah wrote again.

HANNAH: Dear Mr. Pope, *[Imploringly]* Please. Yours truly, Hannah Owen.

HENRY: Dear Mrs. Owen, *[Angrily]* No, goddammit, and if you don't stop this business and get the hell out of my life, I'm going to notify the police. *[Cordially]* Sincerely, Henry Pope.

HANNAH: Dear Mr. Pope, And so your answer is still no. Oh, can you imagine how sad I am? Now I am the one who is disheartened. Never mind. I will try to accept it, as I have no alternative. I shall not be bothering you and your wife again. You can relax. I can't resist saying one more time, although it doesn't matter anymore, that *I* was the owner of the heart. It was mine to give. But that is all water over the dam. Now may I ask you for a much smaller favor? I would like to have a snapshot of you for my scrapbook. Chalk it up to foolish sentiment. Thank you and goodbye. Yours truly, Hannah Owen.

IVY LOU: Hannah, you've been moping around the house for three weeks now. And you're smoking again! Please try and pull yourself together. It was a lousy idea in the first place. What's going to be the end of it?

HANNAH: I don't know, Ivy Lou, I really don't know.

NARRATOR: And then, there it was, lying at the bottom of her mailbox. Hannah scooped it up and held it to her breast, opening it only after she was back in the kitchen, sitting at the table. There was no letter, only the picture.

HANNAH: *[As if talking to Sam]* Oh, Sam, he sent it. He looks so much older than thirty-three. Even with that baseball cap shading his face, I can see he looks very grim indeed. This man has suffered. The picture must have been taken before the operation, for surely he looks healthier now. But he sent it, Sam, he sent it. The heart is working!

NARRATOR: Hannah waited exactly two weeks before she answered. It wasn't easy.

HANNAH: Dear Mr. Pope, Thank you so much for the photo. I have put it in my scrapbook. My friend, Ivy Lou, who is an actuary, has calculated that your face occupies 2.1% of the picture, and with the cap, you are a bit hard to make out. But still. I like your backyard, is it? Are those azaleas on the right of the oak you are leaning against? I have a live oak in my backyard too. Sincerely yours, Hannah Owen.

NARRATOR: Six weeks later, another letter arrived.

HENRY: Dear Mrs. Owen, My wife Inez will be in Little Rock visiting her parents on the weekend of October 20th. If you still want to come, I don't see why not, so long as you just stay for one hour. I will expect you at the house at 10 : 00 Saturday morning. You know where it is, I'm sure. Yours truly, Henry Pope.

HANNAH: You see, Ivy Lou, you see!

IVY LOU: I wouldn't drive if I were you. Not wound as tight as you are. Why, you're as nervous as a bride! See if there's a bus.

NARRATOR: The bus arrived in Avery on Saturday, October 20, at 9 : 30 that morning. Hannah took a cab to 8 Orchard Road. At precisely 10 : 00, she unlatched the front gate and walked up to the door, but before she could ring the bell, the door opened halfway.

[Both Henry and Hannah are very nervous during these next exchanges.]

HENRY: Come in. Excuse the darkness, but I figured I'd keep the drapes drawn. No need to call attention.

HANNAH: Oh, of course. Mr. Pope . . . er, Henry, you look much younger than in the photo you sent me. Very healthy and trim.

HENRY: Yes, well, that was taken before the . . . well . . . before I got better. I lost some weight, too, almost twenty pounds.

NARRATOR: Hannah could see that he was as nervous as she was.

HENRY: Please come with me. We'll go into the den.

HANNAH: Thank you.

HENRY: *[He's not sure how to proceed. He is awkward and not a little uncomfortable.]* It's your show, how do you want me? I suppose you want my T-shirt off. Here.

HANNAH: *[Seeing the deep purple scar on his chest and muttering]* Oh, my. It's quite a scar.

HENRY: Yes, but there's no pain or anything. *[Awkward pause]* Well, how do you want me? Come on, let's get this over with.

HANNAH: Best, I think, for you to lie flat on the sofa. I'll sit on the edge and lean over.

HENRY: Where's your stethoscope?

HANNAH: I don't have a stethoscope.

HENRY: How are you going to listen to my heart without a stethoscope?

HANNAH: They didn't always have them. I'm going to listen with my ear. I have very acute hearing.

HENRY: Well, I don't know . . . oh, it's all right, just go ahead.

NARRATOR: Hannah bent her head, lowering it slowly to Henry's chest. When her cheek touched his skin, she could feel him wince. Hannah closed her eyes and gave herself up to the labor of listening. As she heard the first dull thump, she thought:

HANNAH: *[It's important that during this part Hannah smiles and we see the relief — not a huge, toothy grin, but a smile of pleasure, of gratitude, of true freedom from the anguish she has been feeling for the past three years.]* Oh, that's Samuel's heart, all right. I could pick it out of a thousand. I could listen forever.

NARRATOR: Hannah lay there listening until her ear and the chest of the man fused into a bridge of flesh, across which marched, one beat after another, the parade of that mighty heart. Her own pulse quieted to match it, beat for beat. It seemed that it was no longer sound that entered and occupied her, but blood that flowed from one to the other, her own blood driven by the heart that lay just beneath the breast whose slow rise and fall she rode as though she were a huddled creature waiting to be born. At last Hannah opened her eyes and raised her head. Never, never had she felt such a sense of consolation and happiness. Had it been a dream? Had she fallen asleep? How long had she been there, listening? Then she saw Henry smiling at her and she thought to herself:

HANNAH: Angels must smile like that.

HENRY: [He speaks more gently now, obviously also very moved by the experience.] You were trembling like a bird. Let me help you up, Hannah.

NARRATOR: Henry followed her to the door.

HENRY: [Tenderly] Will you want to come again, Hannah?

NARRATOR: As she stepped out into the light of day, the splendor still singing in her ears, Hannah turned back to Henry and smiled.

HANNAH: No, there will be no need.

END

QUESTIONS FOR DISCUSSION

What is Hannah going through? How will her "wound be healed," as she says, by listening to Sam's heart one more time?

Is Ivy Lou right that Hannah's desire to find the recipient of Sam's heart and listening to Sam's heart one more time is "in the grossest ill taste"? What is Ivy Lou's role in the story?

Why did Hannah stop visiting Sam's grave after going to the butcher? Why is she so confused about whether Sam is alive or dead? Is her confusion understandable?

Why does Hannah react so strongly to words like "harvest" and "transplantation"? Are these words appropriate for the process of removing organs from the newly dead and inserting them into a living person? Hannah makes the transplantation process seem almost ghoulish, especially when she uses words like "dismemberment" and "evisceration." Is it?

Given the pain and other problems Hannah must deal with because of the supposed good deed of donating her husband's organs, should organ transplantation be banned or should the rules about confidentiality and anonymity of donors and recipients be adjusted to allow donors and recipients to know each other? Could the physicians and other members of the transplant team have handled the donation of Sam's organs better?

Did Hannah do anything wrong in the way she tracked down the Popes, or was it justifiable?

Did Inez and Henry Pope respond appropriately to Hannah's initial request and repeated barrage of letters? Should Henry Pope have relented as he did, or should he have stood firm in his refusal?

What have Inez and Henry Pope gone through during Henry's illness, wait for an organ, surgery, and recovery? Do they owe anything to Hannah?

Are there sexual innuendoes in the story? Why did Henry Pope wait until his wife was out of town to fulfill Hannah's request? Should she have used a stethoscope to listen to the heart?

What is the impact of organ transplantation on donors' loved ones and on recipients and their loved ones?

Does the ending of the story justify Hannah's quest and the violation of the Popes' confidentiality and privacy?

Is this the end of the story? What do you imagine happened afterward? Are there possible negative consequences of uniting organ donors and recipients and their families?

Is this story's occasional wry humor too irreverent or offensive given the gravity of the issues raised?

Is the title apt? How does the author make use of the many meanings of the word "heart" in writing this story? Would titling the story after any other body organ work? Why?

The Enemy

PEARL S. BUCK

Adapted for Readers' Theater by Ann Bean

CAST

Yumi (pronounced "yoomee"), a female servant
Dr. Sadao Hoki (Sadao) (pronounced "sadow")
Hana Hoki, wife to Sadao (Hana)
Sailor
Old General (General)

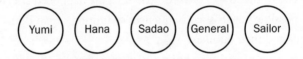

NOTES

When the script says "[To audience]" *readers may look at the audience; when it says* "[To _____ (naming another character)]" *or gives no directions, the reader should use offstage focus.*

YUMI: *[To audience]* I am Yumi. The story you are about to hear took place in Japan during the time of the Great War that devastated my country. It is my privilege to serve in the house of Dr. Sadao Hoki.

SADAO: *[To audience]* My house is built on a spot of the Japanese coast where as a little boy I often played. My house is set upon rocks well above a narrow beach outlined with bent pines. As a boy, I climbed the pines, supporting myself on my bare feet, as I had seen men do in the South Seas when they climbed for coconuts. My father had taken me often to the islands of those seas, and he always said to me, "Those islands yonder, they are the steppingstones to the future for Japan." "Where shall we step from them?" I would ask, and he would always answer, "Who knows? Who can limit our future? It depends on what we make it."

YUMI: *[To audience]* Sadao took this into his mind as he did everything his father said. His father spent infinite pains upon Sadao, his only son. Sadao's education was his father's chief concern. For this reason, he sent Sadao at the age of twenty-two to America to learn all that could be learned of surgery and medicine. He had come back at thirty, and before his father died he had seen Sadao become famous not only as a surgeon but as a scientist.

At the time of the story I am about to tell you, Sadao was perfecting a discovery that would render wounds entirely clean. For that reason, he had not been sent abroad with the troops, but was kept at home to continue his work. Also, the old General whom Sadao was treating was in some slight danger of needing an operation, and for this possibility Sadao was also being kept in Japan.

HANA: *[To audience]* I am Hana, wife of Sadao. My husband met me in America, where I was also a student. We met at the house of an American professor who was eager to do something for foreign students, and, although he and his wife were boring people, we accepted their kindness.

SADAO: *[To audience]* When I met Hana, I felt that I would love her if it were at all possible, but I waited to fall in love with her until I was sure she was Japanese. My father would never have received her unless she had been pure in her race. We finished our work at school and came home to Japan. When my father saw her, the marriage was arranged in the old Japanese way, although Hana and I had talked everything over beforehand. That was many years ago, but even now I often wonder whom I could have married if I had not met Hana.

YUMI: *[To audience]* The story that I have to tell you began several years after Sadao and Hana had married. Their youngest child was only three months old. It was my job to care for them. I loved their children as my own, and my master and mistress as well. That evening, Dr. and

Mrs. Hoki stood on the veranda, she in her blue kimono with her arm through his. She laid her cheek against his arm. It was at this moment that both of them saw something black come out of the mists. It was a man. He was flung up out of the ocean — flung, it seems, to his feet by a breaker. He staggered a few steps, his body outlined against the mist, his arms above his head. Then the curled mists hid him again.

HANA: *[To Sadao]* Sadao, who is that?

YUMI: *[To audience]* She dropped Sadao's arm and they both leaned over the railing of the veranda. Now they saw him again. The man was on his hands and knees crawling. They saw him fall on his face and lie there. They moved quickly down the steps toward him.

SADAO: *[From now on, characters will be in dialogue with each other unless noted otherwise.]* A fisherman perhaps, washed from his boat. He is wounded. *[Pause as he looks closely]* Let me try to turn him so we can see . . .

HANA: *[Horrified]* Oh! He is a white man!

SADAO: *[Slowly, wonderingly]* Yes . . . his yellow hair . . . not cut for many weeks it would seem . . . beard. . . . He is unconscious, but, see, here is his wound . . . it bleeds freshly. And the edges of the wound — gunpowder. It would appear that he was shot but the bullet was not removed. In the water, he has been struck by a rock and the wound has reopened. It is bad luck for him.

HANA: Oh, how he is bleeding!

SADAO: What shall we do with this man? *[Thoughtfully]* I can pack the wound with the seaweed around us. Hana? *[As she hands seaweed to him]* Thank you. See? he moans, but even the pain cannot awaken him. He is in a bad way indeed. *[Pause, then talking to himself]* The best thing that we could do would be to put him back in the sea.

HANA: *[Anxiously]* Yes, undoubtedly that would be best.

SADAO: If we sheltered a white man in our house we could be arrested, and if we turn him over as a prisoner, he would certainly die.

HANA: The kindest thing would be to put him back into the sea. What . . . is he?

SADAO: There is something about him that looks American. His cap has some writing on it . . . *[Reading]* It says "U.S. Navy." A sailor from an American warship. He is a prisoner of war!

HANA: He has escaped! That is why he is wounded.

SADAO: Shot . . . in the back.

HANA: Come, are we able to put him back into the sea?

SADAO: If I am able, are you?

HANA: *[Considering]* No. . . . But if you can do it alone . . .

SADAO: *[Hesitating]* The strange thing is, that if he were whole, I could turn him over to the police without difficulty. I care nothing for him. He is my enemy. All Americans are my enemy. And he is a common fellow. You see how foolish his face is. But since he is wounded . . .

HANA: *[Hana finishes his sentence after a moment.]* . . . you also cannot throw him back to the sea. Then there is only one thing to do. We must carry him into the house.

SADAO: But the servants?

HANA: We must simply tell them that we intend to give him to the police — as indeed, we must, Sadao. We must think of the children and your position. It would endanger all of us if we did not give this man over as a prisoner of war.

SADAO: Certainly. I would not think of doing anything else. Here, help me lift him.

HANA: *[Surprised]* He is so light. He looks like a skeleton, Sadao.

SADAO: Yes, Hana. We will put him in the empty bedroom that was my father's before he died.

HANA: Be careful. Don't let his arms swing and bruise against the door.

SADAO: Put him down gently now. Father's room has not been used for so long — he will disturb no one here.

HANA: There. And there is still an old quilt in the cupboard — the flowered one with the white lining. I'll put it over him. *[Hana pauses as she starts to throw quilt over him and murmurs]* But, he is so dirty!

SADAO: Yes, he had better be washed. If you fetch hot water I will wash him.

HANA: *[Alarmed, repulsed]* I cannot bear for you to touch him! We shall have to tell the servants he is here. I will tell Yumi. She can leave the children for a few minutes and she can wash him.

SADAO: Let it be so. You tell Yumi and I will tell the others. He is very pale and his pulse is very faint. He will die unless he is operated on. The question is whether he will not die anyway.

HANA: Don't try to save him. What if he should live?

SADAO: What if he should die?

HANA: You mean die from the operation?

SADAO: Yes. At any rate, something must be done with him and first he must be washed.

HANA: I will bring Yumi.

SADAO: And I will tell the other servants.

HANA: Yumi! Come with me. Please see that there is an injured man here. He is a white man. He must be an escaped prisoner. Dr. Hoki wishes for you to wash him.

YUMI: *[Alarmed]* I have never washed a white man and I will not wash so dirty a one now.

HANA: *[Firmly]* You will do what your master commands you.

YUMI: *[Stubbornly]* My master ought not to command me to wash the enemy.

HANA: You understand we only want to bring him to his senses so that we can turn him over as a prisoner?

YUMI: I will have nothing to do with it. *[Upset]* I am a poor person and it is not my business.

HANA: *[Gently, seeing Yumi's distress]* I understand. You may return to your own work. *[Muttering to herself]* Stupid Yumi. Is this anything but a man? And a wounded helpless man! *[Resignedly]* Then I will wash him myself. *[Repulsed — by the white man, by the dirt, by the situation]* Oh, my, so much dirt.

SADAO: I am back.

HANA: *[Hana sees Sadao with his surgeon's bag and is alarmed by what it means.]* Your surgeon's bag! And you have put on your surgeon's coat. You have decided to operate!

SADAO: Yes. Fetch towels.

HANA: *[Reluctantly obeying. No disrespect is shown — this is a relationship based on the old Japanese ways.]* Yes, Sadao.

SADAO: Now help me to turn him so I can wash his back.

HANA: Oh! He is bleeding so. The mat is ruined! Yumi would not wash him. She was frightened.

SADAO: Did *you* wash him then?

HANA: Yes . . . he is so young, Sadao. No more than seventeen.

SADAO: The other servants are as frightened as Yumi. They said I should not heal a white man . . . that the white man ought to die. They are afraid if I heal what the gun did and what the sea did that they will take revenge on us. *[Thoughtfully]* You will have to give the anesthetic if he needs it.

HANA: I? But never have I done that!

SADAO: *[Impatient, but not angry]* It is easy enough . . . *[Examining the wounds]* The bullet is still here. I wonder how deep this rock wound is. If it is not too deep it may be that I can get the bullet. But the bleeding is not superficial. He has lost much blood.

HANA: *[Faltering at the sight of the probing and blood]* Oh, Sadao. I cannot watch.

SADAO: Hana, you mustn't faint. If I stop now the man will surely die.

HANA: *[Faintly]* I think I am going to be sick.

SADAO: *[Firmly but not ferociously]* Then leave, Hana. Get sick if you must. But you must pull yourself together then. I need your assistance. *[Speaking to himself then]* There is no reason under heaven why he should live.

SAILOR: *[A soft cry]* Oh . . . oh. *[or "Ah . . . ah." Work this out so it is not comical or too forceful — it is an unconscious stirring.]*

SADAO: Groan if you like, American. I am not doing this for my own pleasure. In fact, I do not know why I am doing it.

HANA: *[Resolved, composed]* I am better and will help you now, Sadao. Where is the anesthetic?

SADAO: That bottle over there. It is well that you came back. This fellow is beginning to stir.

HANA: How shall I do this?

SADAO: Simply saturate the cotton and hold it near his nostrils. When he breathes badly, move it away a little.

HANA: Sadao, what are these marks on his neck. Oh . . . scars . . . terrible red scars! Are the stories of torture true then, Sadao?

SADAO: *[Lost in his work now, Sadao does not respond to her. He speaks as if to himself.]* There it is. So near the kidney but not penetrating it. I knew it would be close. American bodies are still put together the same way as Japanese ones. And I was taught well. What did he always say, my old professor of anatomy? — "Ignorance of the human body is the surgeon's cardinal sin, sirs!" He shouted it, every year the same words — "To operate without as complete knowledge of the body as if you had made it — anything less than that is murder." *[Sadao laughs softly to himself as he remembers. He addresses his next words to the American.]* Yes, I know your body, American, and you are lucky. It is not quite to the kidney, my friend. *[Hearing himself say "friend," he looks up in surprise and says the next words to himself again.]* "Friend" — already as if he were one of my own patients — well . . . *[He tenses as he peers closely at his work and speaks aloud again.]* There. Fast and neat . . . it is out. *[He looks up with pride and relief.]*

SAILOR: *[Low moan]* Ohhh . . . *[Muttering]* Guts . . . they got . . . my guts.

HANA: *[Alarmed]* Sadao!

SADAO: *[Consolingly to Hana]* Shhhhh. It is over. No more anesthetic. Please bring me the bandages. I will stitch and dress the wound. *[Speaking to himself]* Surely I do not want this man to live.

HANA: *[Not hearing him]* I'm sorry, Sadao, I did not hear the last words you said.

SADAO: Nothing, Hana, nothing. This man will live in spite of all.

YUMI: *[To audience]* The young man slept for a very long time. Dr. Hoki checked on him often and with as much care as if he had been one of our own countrymen. We servants were frightened and refused to go near the room of our enemy, even when my mistress asked us for simple things like blankets or towels. So she tended him herself. At last he awakened.

SAILOR: *[Awakening]* Wha . . . ? But who are you?

HANA: Don't be afraid.

SAILOR: How come . . . you speak English?

HANA: I was a long time in America.

SAILOR: *[Very weak]* Where . . . ? What am I doing . . . ?

HANA: Do not try to speak. You must eat. I will help you. Soon you will be strong.

YUMI: *[To audience]* For the next three days the white man was in my master's house — unknown to the authorities. The other servants and I grew daily more watchful. The cook and the gardener, who had been with Dr. Hoki's family since he was a small boy, were as courteous and as careful as ever, but their eyes were cold when they looked upon the master or mistress. Still, we could not betray him to the authorities.

SADAO: *[To Sailor]* American! What are you doing up? Lie down! Do you want to die? You may kill yourself if you do this sort of thing.

SAILOR: What are you going to do to me? Are you going to hand me over?

SADAO: I do not know myself what I shall do with you. I ought, of course, to give you to the police. You are a prisoner of war.

SAILOR: I am . . .

SADAO: *[Interrupting him]* No! Do not tell me anything. Do not even tell me your name unless I ask it. Now you must rest. I will return later.

HANA: Sadao, I have been waiting out here to speak to you. Yumi tells me the servants feel they cannot stay if we hide this man here any longer. They are saying that you and I were so long in America that we have forgotten to think of our own country first. They think we like Americans.

SADAO: *[Angrily]* It is not true! Americans are our enemies. But I have been trained not to let a man die if I can help it.

HANA: The servants cannot understand that.

SADAO: No. And I can understand why it is hard for them. I was brought up as they were.

YUMI: *[To audience]* The gardener was saying, "My master's son knows very well what he ought to do" — see, he even spoke of the old man long dead as his "master" still. "When the man was so near death," he said, "why did he not let him bleed?" And the old cook said that the young master is so proud of his skill to save life . . . *[say next five words with Hana]* that he saves any life.

HANA: *[Speaking the last words along with Yumi, but addressing her husband]* that he saves any life. Sadao, they speak of these things when they know I am near enough to hear them. And I know they are right. But there is some small place inside of me that is proud that you saved this life,

Sadao. Today when I took him his breakfast, before I could leave the room, the man said:

SAILOR: My name is Tom.

HANA: I did not speak, only bowed and left the room. But as I left, I could see a look of fear in his eyes. Oh, Sadao! He is a great trouble in this house!

SADAO: Yes, Hana, I know what you are saying. Only yesterday when I had removed the last few stitches, I went to my office and began typing a report to the chief of police about how an escaped prisoner had been washed up on the shore in front of my house. But I stopped and hid the unfinished letter.

YUMI: *[To audience]* On the seventh day, we servants left Dr. Hoki's house. We cried many tears. For the cook and the gardener had served Dr. Hoki since he was a child, and I had served his children since their births. I ran back to tell my mistress that I would return if the baby missed me too much. But I could see in her eyes that she would not send for me, no matter how hard the baby cried.

HANA: Sadao, why is it we cannot see clearly what we ought to do? Even the servants see more clearly than we do. Why are we different from other Japanese?

SADAO: *[In thought]* I have no answer, Hana. I must see my patient now. *[To Sailor]* American, today you may get up on your feet. I want you to stay up only five minutes at a time. Tomorrow you may try it twice as long. It would be well that you get back your strength as quickly as possible.

SAILOR: Okay. *[Unsure of what is to come]* I feel I ought to thank you, Doctor, for having saved my life.

SADAO: *[Coolly]* Don't thank me too early. I will leave you now. Remember — only five minutes.

HANA: *[Calling]* Sadao! Sadao!

SADAO: What is it, Hana?

HANA: A messenger from the palace came for you. I was so frightened! I thought they'd come to arrest you! But it is the old General. He is sick and you are needed. I was so relieved and without thinking I said to the messenger, "Oh, is that all?" He looked fiercely at me and said, "All? Is that not enough?!" I told him it certainly was and that I was very sorry the General was not well. Forgive me, Sadao.

SADAO: No, Hana, it is you who should forgive me. I must get rid of this man for your sake and the children's sake. Somehow, I must get rid of him. But now, I must go to the General.

YUMI: *[To audience]* And so the Doctor went to the palace to serve the old General. I know this is so because when the old General called for Dr. Hoki, word of this spread quickly. For both men were treasures of Japan.

SADAO: And so, Excellency, that is the whole story of the American.

GENERAL: Of course, I understand fully. But that is because I once took a degree in Princeton. So few Japanese have.

SADAO: I care nothing for the man, but having operated on him with such success . . .

GENERAL: Yes, yes. It only makes me feel you are more indispensable to me. Evidently you can save anyone — you are so skilled. You say you think I can stand one more attack as I have had today?

SADAO: Not more than one.

GENERAL: Then certainly I can allow nothing to happen to you. *[Decidedly]* You cannot be arrested. Suppose you were condemned to death and the next day I had to have my operation?

SADAO: There are other surgeons, Excellency.

GENERAL: None I trust. *[Sarcastically]* The best ones have been trained by Germans and would consider the operation successful even if I died. I do not care for their point of view. It seems a pity that we cannot better combine the German ruthlessness with the American sentimentality. Then you could turn your prisoner over to execution and yet I could be sure you would not murder me while I was unconscious. *[He laughs.]* As a Japanese, could you not combine these two foreign elements?

SADAO: *[Smiling, thinking General has an unusual sense of humor]* I am not quite sure, but for your sake I would be willing to try, Excellency.

GENERAL: I had rather not be the test case. *[Irritably]* It is very unfortunate that this man should have washed up on your doorstep.

SADAO: *[Gently]* I feel it so myself.

GENERAL: It would be best if he could be quietly killed. Not by you, but by someone who does not know him. I have my own private assassins. Suppose I send two of them to your house tonight — or better, any night. You need know nothing about it. It is now warm — what would be more natural than that you should leave the outer partition of the white man's room open to the garden while he sleeps?

SADAO: Certainly it would be very natural. In fact, it is so left every night.

GENERAL: Good. They are very capable assassins — they make no noise and they know the trick of inward bleeding. If you like, I can even have them remove the body.

SADAO: That perhaps would be best. I would prefer that my wife does not know about the assassins. If the man is gone, she will think he has escaped.

GENERAL: Yes, of course. Think of it no more.

SADAO: Thank you, Excellency. I'll leave you now to rest.

YUMI: *[To audience]* I could not help but worry about the Doctor and Mrs. Hoki. How would he deal with the white man, who surely must be well by now? For I had not been called back by my mistress and I knew she would send for me when the enemy was gone.

SADAO: *[To Sailor]* What is this, American?! Who gave you permission to leave your room?

SAILOR: I was only going into the garden. *[Good naturedly]* I'm not used to asking permission. *[Brightly]* Gosh, I feel pretty good again! But will the muscles on this side always feel stiff?

SADAO: Stiff? Is it so? *[Now as doctor to patient, not enemy to enemy]* Now I thought I had provided against that. Let me see, massage may do it if exercise does not.

SAILOR: It won't bother me much. Say Doctor, I've got to say something to you. If I hadn't met a Jap like you — well, I wouldn't be alive today. I know that.

SADAO: *[Sadao says nothing, but the reader might do a small bow of the head here, as the Japanese do — nothing huge, just a slight nod with downcast eyes]*

SAILOR: Sure, I know that. I guess if all the Japs were like you, there wouldn't have been a war.

SADAO: *[Stiffly]* Perhaps. *[As doctor to patient again]* And now I think you had better go back to bed. Let me help you. Goodnight.

SAILOR: Goodnight. And thanks again.

YUMI: The next morning . . .

HANA: Is something wrong, Sadao? Why did you rise so early?

SADAO: I slept badly last night. I woke many times. There seemed to be footsteps outside, twigs snapping. Like someone was carrying something across our garden.

HANA: Maybe he has escaped?

SADAO: No, I have just checked his room. He is sleeping soundly. He is almost well to sleep like that.

HANA: *[The question is a familiar one by now. Hana speaks almost automatically.]* What shall we do with him?

SADAO: *[Placating but kind]* I know. I must decide in a day or two. *[To himself]* Tonight, then, surely.

YUMI: That evening . . .

HANA: The wind is strong tonight, Sadao.

SADAO: Yes, I am sorry that it has woken you, too, Hana. Hear how it whistles through the branches and the very walls of our house. As if someone were calling out.

HANA: Do you suppose we should check on the American? We left the outer partition of his room open ought we not to go and close it?

SADAO: *[Quickly]* No! *[Catching himself, and speaking with less outward show of alarm]* It is not cold, and the wind is blowing toward the sea and not from it. Besides, he is able now to do it for himself.

YUMI: The following morning . . .

SAILOR: Hi! That was some blow last night, wasn't it. It's amazing how strong your houses are. Seems like they'd just fold up and fly off.

SADAO: *[Hardly hearing him]* Yes . . . I'm glad you were not uncomfortable. *[Speaking to himself]* Tonight, then. It must be tonight.

YUMI: That night . . .

HANA: What was that noise? Oh, it has frightened the baby. I will go.

SADAO: Don't go. Don't go!

HANA: Sadao, what is the matter with you?

YUMI: The following morning . . .

SAILOR: *[Joyously]* I feel great.

SADAO: *[With total exhaustion — he can't take another night of this. He nods his head.]* You are well. *[Dropping his voice]* You are so well that I think if I put my boat on the shore tonight with food and extra clothing in it, you might be able to row to that little island not far from the coast. It is so near the coast, that it has not been worth fortifying. Nobody lives on it because in storm it is submerged. But this is not the season of the storm. You could live there until you saw a Korean fishing boat pass by. They pass quite near the island because the water is many fathoms deep there.

SAILOR: *[Slowly comprehending]* Do I have to?

SADAO: I think so. You understand — it is not hidden that you are here.

SAILOR: *[Nodding, simply]* Okay.

SADAO: I will go now to prepare things for you. There will be no moon tonight. After it is dark, I will come back. Until later, then.

HANA: Yumi was here today, Sadao. She cried over the baby. She misses him so.

SADAO: The servants will come back as soon as the foreigner is gone. Now I have some work to do. Then I will look in on him once more tonight. You need not bother again, Hana.

HANA: *[Understanding that he is telling her he is taking care of the situation]* Thank you, Sadao. I will go and put the baby to bed.

SADAO: *[To Sailor]* It is ready, American.

SAILOR: I realize you are saving my life again.

SADAO: Not at all. It is only inconvenient to have you here any longer. Take this flashlight. If your food runs out before you catch a boat, signal me two flashes at the same instant the sun drops over the horizon. Do not signal in darkness, for it will be seen. If you are all right, but still there, signal me once. You will find fish easy to catch but you must eat them raw. A fire would be seen.

SAILOR: Okay.

SADAO: Go quickly now.

YUMI: We returned to our master's house and the white man was never spoken of. I burned sulphur in the guest room to get the white man's smell out of it. The gardener was cross because he had got behind with his chrysanthemums. The following week, Dr. Hoki was called to the General's, where he performed an emergency operation. He attended the General daily and after a week, the General began to get his strength back.

GENERAL: You say the man escaped?

SADAO: Yes, Excellency.

GENERAL: *[Remembering]* The prisoner, did I not promise you I would kill him for you?

SADAO: You did, Excellency.

GENERAL: *[Flustered]* Well, well, so I did. *[Making excuses for forgetting]* But you see, I was suffering a good deal. The truth is, I thought of nothing but myself. *[He is ashamed.]* In short, I forgot my promise to you.

SADAO: I wondered, Your Excellency.

GENERAL: It was certainly careless of me. But you understand it was not lack of patriotism or dereliction of duty. *[Anxiously]* If the matter should come out you would understand, wouldn't you?

SADAO: Certainly, Your Excellency. I can swear to your loyalty, Excellency, and to your zeal against the enemy.

GENERAL: You are a good man! *[Relieved]* You will be rewarded.

YUMI: For many nights my master would stand on the veranda and gaze at the sunset, as if he was looking for something — as if he expected to see something. And then one evening as I was preparing the baby for bed, I saw both my master and mistress looking down at the sea. They spoke in low tones.

SADAO: *[Sincerely, from the heart, without malice]* Having the white man here made me remember how difficult it was for me to find a place to live in America when I was a student. The Americans were full of prejudice and each day was a test. Only at the university did I find some acceptance, but even there it was never complete. I knew I was superior to them and yet I was always in a position of gratitude it seemed. I believe in this war, Hana. I still find white people repulsive. That young sailor — so colorless, skin almost transparent.

HANA: *[Gently]* He is gone now, Sadao.

SADAO: Strange . . . I wonder why I could not kill him?

END

QUESTIONS FOR DISCUSSION

Why did Sadao act as he did? Did he do the right thing? How would you characterize Sadao?

What is the issue or conflict in this story? Which is more important in your opinion: loyalty to one's country or one's duty as a physician/health professional to heal the ailing? Does the role of the physician change in wartime?

Why did Yumi and the other servants act as they did? Were they justified in their behavior? Do differences in class or education among the characters play a role in the story? Why did the servants not go to the authorities?

How did Hana react to the situation at first? What is her role in the story?

To whom or to what does the title of the story refer?

Do racial or ethnic attitudes play a role in the story? Do you think race influenced Sadao's decision to treat the American? Did it influence the kind of care he gave him? How do you think pride factored into Sadao's decision to attempt surgery and save the American?

Why did Sadao not want to know the sailor's name?

Do you think the General really forgot to send assassins to kill the sailor? What is the role of the General in the story?

What message do you take away from this story? What does the story say about bias in medicine?

The Doctors of Hoyland

ARTHUR CONAN DOYLE

Adapted for Readers' Theater by Gregory A. Watkins

CAST

Elspeth

Dr. James Ripley (Dr. Ripley)

Thomas

Mrs. Crowder (Crowder)

Rachel Crews (Rachel)

Dr. Verrinder Smith (Dr. Smith)

William Ripley (William)

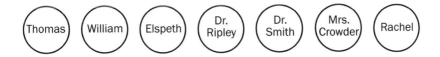

NOTES

Gregory Watkins, the adapter of this story, created two humorous characters, maids to Drs. Ripley and Smith, who eavesdrop at their employers' keyholes and gossip with townspeople, to serve as vehicles for telling the story.

Elspeth acts as both narrator and story character. When she is speaking as narrator, indicated in the script by "[To audience]," she should look directly at the audience and talk conversationally and engagingly. When interacting with other characters in the story, indicated in the script by "[To ——— (name of character)]," she should use offstage focus, as should all the other characters.

Thomas is a bit slow on the uptake. If necessary, one person can play both

William Ripley *and* Thomas, *and one person can play both* Rachel *and* Mrs. Crowder.

The name of the Scottish city Edinburgh is pronounced as if spelled "Edinboro." The Lancet *is a British medical journal.*

ELSPETH: *[To audience]* Good evening. It has fallen to me, the good Lord alone knows why, as I hate to talk about other people and their affairs without their knowledge, to relate to you the story of Doctors Ripley and Smith, and the events that befell them here in the village of Hoyland, in the north of Hampshire, in the year of our Lord, eighteen-hundred-and-ninety-four. To be completely forthright, some of the story I got secondhand (though on very good authority), but the most of it I saw with my own two eyes, or heard with my own two ears, and not through keyholes either, lest you be thinking that way. It is not uncommon for me, in the course of my duties as housekeeper to Dr. Ripley, to pass by his . . . oh dear! I forgot to introduce myself. Please forgive me. My name is . . .

DR. RIPLEY: *[As if calling from another room]* ELSPETH.

ELSPETH: Uhm, Elspeth. And that was Dr. Ripley.

DR. RIPLEY: ELSPETH!!

ELSPETH: *[Now in same room] [To Dr. Ripley]* Yes, Doctor.

DR. RIPLEY: Elspeth, would you ask Thomas to ready a carriage, please?

ELSPETH: *[To Dr. Ripley]* Yes, Doctor. *[To audience]* Thomas is Doctor's groom and carriage driver. He's a good enough fellow, though a bit slow-witted and given to spirits.

DR. RIPLEY: *[Impatient]* Elspeth!

ELSPETH: *[To Dr. Ripley and Thomas]* Yes, Doctor. Thomas! *[To audience]* Doctor is usually so patient, except when he's in a hurry. *[To Thomas]* Thomas!

THOMAS: Yes'm.

ELSPETH: Thomas, Dr. Ripley has asked that you ready a carriage. He has a call to make.

THOMAS: Yes'm.

ELSPETH: And be quick about it.

THOMAS: Yes'm.

DR. RIPLEY: Elspeth, Thomas, good morning.

ELSPETH: Good morning, Doctor.

THOMAS: Morning.

DR. RIPLEY: I have to call on the Widow Crowder this morning, Thomas. One of her daughters has taken sick. Prepare a carriage and I'll meet you at the stable.

THOMAS: Yes, sir.

DR. RIPLEY: Elspeth, should anyone call while I'm out, tell them I'll be back this afternoon.

ELSPETH: Yes, Doctor. *[Pause] [To audience]* Mrs. Crowder's daughters usually take sick closer to supper time, if you catch my meaning, and they usually recover the moment Dr. Ripley arrives. Doctor, being a gentleman, has always attributed these recoveries to the course of nature, and I suppose nature is involved, though not, I think, in the way Doctor means. You see, Mrs. Crowder's husband passed away seven years ago, but not before he had blessed her with four lovely (in her estimation if no one else's) daughters. Four daughters Mrs. Crowder has made it her life's work to marry off, and marry well. Thus far, she has been successful with the two eldest, and has decided that Doctor is the leading candidate for one of the two remaining. I have tried, on a number of occasions, to deflect her, as I know Doctor has no interest in marrying at this time, but to no avail. She has a well-developed ability to ignore what she doesn't want to hear. Just last Wednesday, at market . . .
[Elspeth and Crowder stand and face at 45-degree angles toward each other so they are talking to opposite corners of the room.]

CROWDER: *[All through her lines, Mrs. Crowder speaks breathlessly and barely allows room for Elspeth's responses.]* Why, Elspeth, how nice to see you again.

ELSPETH: Good morning, ma'am.

CROWDER: How are you, Elspeth?

ELSPETH: Quite well, ma'am.

CROWDER: And Dr. Ripley?

ELSPETH: Oh, he's very busy, and well.

CROWDER: And such a fine young man. I tell you, Elspeth, when old Dr. Ripley passed on, I think everyone in this town was afraid young Dr. Ripley would move away, to a city, perhaps. After all, he is young, and very handsome, and I'm sure he could be a success anywhere he went, but he stayed, and I'm sure we are all very grateful he did.

ELSPETH: Yes, ma'am.

CROWDER: I'm sure that's why the good folk of Hoyland have always ignored the rival doctors who have set up here since young Dr. Ripley took up his father's practice. I daresay none of the newcomers took more than a shilling or two of Dr. Ripley's custom, nor did they deserve even that.

ELSPETH: Indeed, ma'am.

CROWDER: No, Dr. Ripley is Hoyland's doctor, and shall remain so as long as he wishes. In fact, all that remains for him is to take a fine young Hoyland girl to wife, and his life will be well finished.

ELSPETH: Doctor has shown no inclination to take a wife, ma'am.

CROWDER: Well, that's because he hasn't met the right girl yet, isn't it? Or, having met her, hasn't recognized her as a proper companion. I can't help but think if he would spend just a little time with Margaret (she's the third eldest of my lovely daughters), that he would see straightaway what a good match they could be.

ELSPETH: Margaret, she's the *tall* one, isn't she?

CROWDER: Not so tall. Certainly no taller than she should be, and such a splendid cook.

ELSPETH: Doctor is so busy, ma'am.

CROWDER: But he is forever shut up in his study. Whatever could keep him so occupied?

ELSPETH: His studies, ma'am. Doctor prides himself on his medical knowledge. Why, at a moment's notice, he can hold forth for hours on some obscure body part or condition or such. There's not a doctor outside London more knowledgeable.

CROWDER: Of course, of course. But he might look to his personal life a bit more closely. It wouldn't do him any harm to look for a little more pleasure from life, and what could give him more pleasure than a loving and devoted wife?

ELSPETH: Yes'm, but he's . . .

CROWDER: *[Interrupting]* Well, I must run. I'm teaching Margaret how to make a three-cheese souffle, and I'd like to have it ready in time for supper. Give my best to Dr. Ripley.

[Both sit.]

ELSPETH: *[To audience]* You see what I mean? You can't get a word in edgewise, and what you do get in, she ignores. And Margaret! I daresay she would be the most likely of Widow Crowder's daughters to get Doctor's attention, but only because he has such a profound affection for horses. At any rate, Doctor has become quite adept at avoiding Mrs. Crowder's ploys, chiefly through extensive practice. Almost every Hoyland girl of marriageable age has been tossed in his path at some time or other, and he has learned to sidestep them rather well. And I really do believe it is because of his love for his medicine. In fact, he is almost fanatical about it. I don't know how many times I have entered his study in the morning, to find journals and papers scattered hither and yon, or some more of those sheep's eyes sent up by the butcher, on which he has been practicing at his art. Really, it is a horrid mess.

[Realizing she has digressed] Oh, I set out to tell you the story of Doctors Ripley and Smith, and so I shall. To begin at the beginning, it was on an afternoon in April, 1894, and Doctor had just returned from a call . . .

DR. RIPLEY: Elspeth, good afternoon.

ELSPETH: *[To Dr. Ripley]* Good afternoon, Doctor.

DR. RIPLEY: It seems I have acquired a new rival.

ELSPETH: Oh?

DR. RIPLEY: Yes, a Dr. Verrinder Smith. He's set up a practice in a new house in lower Hoyland.

ELSPETH: Really? Do you know him?

DR. RIPLEY: No, and I doubt I should forget a name like Verrinder. Very unusual. Let's see if he's listed in the current medical directory. Where did I put that . . . ?

ELSPETH: Here, Doctor.

DR. RIPLEY: Thank you, Elspeth. Now let's see, Smith, *[pause]* Smith. Ah, here it is, "Verrinder Smith, M.D."

ELSPETH: *[Pause]* What's it say?

DR. RIPLEY: Very impressive. Very superb degrees. Studied with distinction at Edinburgh, Paris, Berlin, Vienna. Awarded a gold medal, and the Lee Hopkins Scholarship for original research, "In recognition of an exhaustive inquiry into the functions of the anterior spinal nerve roots."

ELSPETH: What does that mean?

DR. RIPLEY: It means he's a superb physician. With an excellent record. But what on earth would such a doctor be doing in a little hamlet like Hoyland?

ELSPETH: Resting?

DR. RIPLEY: One needn't hang a shingle to rest, Elspeth; no, he must have some reason . . .

ELSPETH: Perhaps he heard about Mrs. Crowder's unwed daughters.

DR. RIPLEY: Elspeth!

ELSPETH: Sorry, Doctor.

DR. RIPLEY: Wait. He has an excellent record in research. Perhaps he's come here to pursue some further inquiries in peace and quiet. Of course, that must be it.

ELSPETH: Then why did he hang a shingle?

DR. RIPLEY: Well, a shingle needn't be an advertisement. I'm sure it is meant to serve as an address. Oh, this is wonderful, Elspeth, simply wonderful!

ELSPETH: How so?

DR. RIPLEY: To have so brilliant a neighbor will be a splendid thing for my own studies. A kindred mind, a steel on which to strike my flint. I shall have to meet him straightaway. I'll pay him a call in the morning.

ELSPETH: Doctor?

DR. RIPLEY: Hmmm??

ELSPETH: Isn't it customary for a new doctor to pay a call upon the older first? As a matter of courtesy?

DR. RIPLEY: Well, yes, but I'm not about to let such a small consideration delay my meeting with such a man for even a day. Ah, Elspeth, this is good news, indeed.

ELSPETH: *[To audience]* And so saying, he dashed off to his study, and re-mained there the rest of the day, not even taking his supper. I had never seen him so excited before, *[pause, sounding suddenly more serious]* nor since. Certainly not since.

> *[Back to more jaunty style]* At any rate, the following afternoon I was again at market, where I chanced to meet Rachel Crews, a young girl of lower Hoyland with aspirations to be a maid . . .

[Both stand and face as in Elspeth's conversation with Mrs. Crowder.]

RACHEL: Miss Elspeth, oh, I have news!

ELSPETH: Now, Rachel, if you think to share some awful bit of gossip with me, you know I don't . . .

RACHEL: *[Interrupting]* Oh, no! no! It's not gossip, well, not really.

ELSPETH: Very well, I'll listen, but only for a moment.

RACHEL: Oh, thank you. Where to begin? Well, as you know, I've been looking for a position as a maid for some time.

ELSPETH: Yes.

RACHEL: Well, earlier this week I found one with the new doctor in town.

ELSPETH: Verrinder Smith?

RACHEL: The same.

ELSPETH: How interesting. Congratulations, that is excellent news.

RACHEL: Oh, that's not my news. Well it is, but it isn't. I mean, my real news concerns Dr. Ripley.

ELSPETH: Dr. Ripley?

RACHEL: Yes. He came to pay a call on Dr. Smith this morning.

ELSPETH: Yes. I knew he had planned to do so.

RACHEL: Well, so he did. I showed him into the consulting room, and took his card in to Dr. Smith, who told me to have Dr. Ripley wait for a moment. When I came back into the consulting room, I could tell Dr. Ripley was well impressed with what he saw there. Dr. Smith's in-struments are all very new and very elaborate. Dr. Ripley looked closely at each of them, and I could see that he was growing more excited with each new discovery. After he had looked at the instruments he went to Dr. Smith's medical library and started staring at the title of each vol-ume, making little noises from time to time, as if he were surprised, or delighted. While he was looking at the library, Dr. Smith came into the consulting room and excused me. I said "good morning" to both the Doctors and left the room, but I stopped outside the door to listen.

ELSPETH: Rachel, I am shocked!!

RACHEL: I couldn't help it.

ELSPETH: Child, I am so disappointed in you. Eavesdropping!

RACHEL: Let me finish, please.

ELSPETH: Very well, the damage is done.

RACHEL: Thank you, thank you, thank you.

ELSPETH: *[Eager to hear the rest of the story]* Go ahead, child, what happened next?

RACHEL: Well, then I heard . . .

[Rachel and Elspeth freeze.]

DR. SMITH: *[Dr. Smith maintains her dignity and decorum throughout this exchange with Dr. Ripley.]* How do you do, Dr. Ripley?

DR. RIPLEY: How do you do, madam? Is your husband out?

DR. SMITH: I'm not married.

DR. RIPLEY: Oh, I beg your pardon! I meant the doctor, Dr. Verrinder Smith.

DR. SMITH: I am Dr. Verrinder Smith.

DR. RIPLEY: *[Flustered]* What? But . . . but I thought . . . you mean . . . the Lee Hopkins prize . . . you?

DR. SMITH: *[Amused by his reaction]* I am sorry to disappoint you.

DR. RIPLEY: You certainly have surprised me.

DR. SMITH: You don't approve of female physicians, then?

DR. RIPLEY: No, I can't say I do.

DR. SMITH: And why not?

DR. RIPLEY: I'd prefer not to discuss it.

DR. SMITH: Oh, but I'm sure you will answer a lady's question.

DR. RIPLEY: Ladies are in danger of losing their privileges when they usurp the place of the other sex. They can't claim both.

DR. SMITH: Why shouldn't a woman earn her bread with her brains?

DR. RIPLEY: I'd prefer not to be led into a discussion, Miss Smith.

DR. SMITH: *Doctor* Smith.

DR. RIPLEY: *Doctor* Smith. Well, if you insist on an answer, I must say no, I do not think medicine is a suitable profession for women, and I have a personal objection to masculine ladies.

DR. SMITH: It seems to me you're begging the question. Of course, if the practice of medicine makes women masculine that would be a considerable deterioration.

DR. RIPLEY: I must go.

DR. SMITH: I'm sorry we can't come to a friendlier conclusion, since we are to be neighbors.

DR. RIPLEY: Good morning, Dr. Smith.

DR. SMITH: It was a singular coincidence that at the instant you called I was reading your paper on "Locomotor Ataxia" in *The Lancet*.

DR. RIPLEY: Oh?

DR. SMITH: Yes, I thought it a very able monograph.

DR. RIPLEY: *[Warming somewhat]* You are too kind.

DR. SMITH: But the views you attribute to Professor Pitres, of Bordeaux, he has repudiated.

DR. RIPLEY: I have his pamphlet of 1890.

DR. SMITH: Here is his pamphlet of 1891. I believe you'll find . . .

DR. RIPLEY: *[Interrupting — flustered again]* Good day, Miss Smith.
[Elspeth and Rachel resume their conversation.]

RACHEL: And Dr. Ripley came out of the office as if he had the devil himself on his tail.

ELSPETH: The devil *her*self, more like. A woman, you say, and a doctor?

RACHEL: The same.

ELSPETH: Well, I'll be. Rachel, don't you dare tell another soul about this exchange between our doctors. If you do, I'll have your tongue out.

RACHEL: Not a soul, Miss Elspeth, I promise. Telling you was quite enough.

ELSPETH: Good girl. Now run along. And remember, not a word. *[Pause]* *[To audience]* And as far as I know, she kept her promise, which makes you the first to hear the story since she told it to me. At any rate, I rushed straight home, and found Doctor in as ill a humor as you might expect. I overheard Doctor talking to Thomas in his study.

DR. RIPLEY: A woman! Damn it, Thomas, a woman!

THOMAS: *[Dully, not quite grasping why Dr. Ripley is so upset]* Is that bad, then?

DR. RIPLEY: Of course it is, Thomas. The rigors of a medical education are a fit trial for a man, and nothing short of a scandal for a woman.

THOMAS: Oh, right.

DR. RIPLEY: You see, Thomas, there are elements of the medical education that are not proper subject matter for the delicate sensibilities of the fairer sex. Why, some of the less vigorous men had trouble with part of the curriculum.

THOMAS: Oh, I see.

DR. RIPLEY: Nor does it end with the education. A practice will bring her into contact with things no proper lady should ever be exposed to. *[Pause]* Elspeth!

ELSPETH: *[To Dr. Ripley]* Uhm, yes, Doctor?

DR. RIPLEY: If you are going to listen at the door you must learn to breathe more softly.

ELSPETH: Yes, Doctor.

DR. RIPLEY: Well, come in, come in.

ELSPETH: Yes, Doctor.

DR. RIPLEY: Even if women are to be doctors, Verrinder Smith seems a very unlikely candidate. She is . . . *[softening briefly]* too young . . . too slender . . . too feminine. Were she not so supercilious, she might even be accounted attractive. *[Back to being upset]* Hardly the sort one would expect to be lancing the boil on a miner's bum!

ELSPETH: Doctor!!

DR. RIPLEY: Excuse me, Elspeth, I'm unsettled.

THOMAS: I'll fetch the carriage.

DR. RIPLEY: What?

THOMAS: You'll be wanting a ride in the country about now.

DR. RIPLEY: I will? Yes, of course.

THOMAS: Meet you at the stable.

DR. RIPLEY: Excellent. And Elspeth, I apologize for my ill humor. A gentleman must maintain his equanimity, even under the most trying circumstances. I do hope you forgive me my outburst.

ELSPETH: Of course, Doctor. Everything's fine. *[To audience]* And so it was . . . *[ironically]* for almost no time at all. You see, Dr. Smith did indeed receive patients — receive them with a skill that made those who had come to her because Doctor Ripley was not available remain with her even when he was. In fact, those she tended were so impressed by the fancy instruments she used, they could speak of nothing else for weeks afterward. And soon there were tangible proofs of her powers. She cured Farmer Eyton's callous ulcer with some sort of ointment. She removed a birthmark from Mrs. Crowder's youngest *lovely* daughter, Eliza, through the use of something called galvanic needles. In a month, Dr. Verrinder Smith was known. In two, she was famous. Nor was her fame lost on Dr. Ripley.

DR. RIPLEY: *[Resignedly]* Is there anyone to see me this morning, Elspeth?

ELSPETH: *[To Dr. Ripley]* No, Doctor.

DR. RIPLEY: I see. *[Bitterly]* I suppose they're all down to see that *unsexed* woman in lower Hoyland.

ELSPETH: I suppose they may be. *[To audience]* And, of course, they were. But as much as the loss of custom galled Dr. Ripley, what galled him more was Dr. Smith's performance of procedures he considered impracticable. Doctor, for all his medical knowledge, was an indifferent surgeon, and sent all his worst cases to London. Dr. Smith, however, had no such weakness, and took everything that came her way. And when she operated on little Alec Turner's club foot, Alec's mother asked Doctor Ripley to act as chloroformist. He was loathe to act as Dr. Smith's assistant, but to refuse would have been cruel, so he accepted. The operation was . . .

DR. RIPLEY: *[Coldly polite]* As masterfully done as I have ever seen, Dr. Smith.

DR. SMITH: *[Assuming the same tone in return]* Thank you, Dr. Ripley.

ELSPETH: And, of course, spread her fame even more widely. Doctor began to detest her. Then, one winter's evening, a groom from Squire Faircastle's came riding down to say that the Squire's daughter had scalded her hand and needed medical help immediately. He had also told Dr. Smith, as the Squire didn't care who came, as long as they came swiftly. Doctor had Thomas ready a carriage instantly and made straightaway for the Squire's keep, hoping to beat Dr. Smith there. Unfortunately, Thomas, in his haste, had neglected to light the carriage's lamps, and, in the dark, failed to negotiate a sharp turn in Basingstoke road. The carriage overturned, throwing Thomas into the road and Doctor into a ditch. When Thomas had recovered sufficiently, he crawled to where Doctor lay, and was immediately sick.

THOMAS: Oh, Lord!

DR. RIPLEY: Damn!

THOMAS: Oh, Doctor! Your bone's poking right through your trouser leg. Oh Lord!

DR. RIPLEY: *[In obvious pain]* Compound fracture. Thomas, get help.

ELSPETH: So Thomas continued to the Squire's afoot, as they were closer to there than to home. Dr. Ripley fainted. When he came to he saw a small page holding a carriage lamp near his injured leg, and a woman, with an open case of polished instruments gleaming in the yellow light, slitting up his trouser with a crooked scissors.

DR. SMITH: *[Sympathetically]* It's all right, Doctor. I am so sorry about this.

DR. RIPLEY: *[Unbelievingly]* You!

DR. SMITH: You can have Dr. Horton tomorrow, but I'm sure you'll allow me to help you tonight.

DR. RIPLEY: Thomas has gone for help.

DR. SMITH: When it comes we can put you in my carriage. More light, John. Oh dear, we shall have laceration unless we reduce this before we move you. Here, take a breath of this chloroform.

ELSPETH: But Dr. Ripley had already fainted again. When he recovered his senses, he found himself in his own bed, with a head like a cannonball and a leg like an iron bar — and Dr. Verrinder Smith in attendance.

DR. SMITH: Well, at last. I kept you under all the way home, for I knew how painful the jolting would be. Your leg is in a good position now, with a strong side splint. I have also ordered a morphia draft for you.

DR. RIPLEY: Thank you.

DR. SMITH: Shall I tell Thomas to ride for Dr. Horton in the morning?

DR. RIPLEY: I'd prefer you continue the case. *[Dryly]* You have the rest of

Hoyland as patients, you know, so you may as well make things complete by having me also.

DR. SMITH: As you wish.

ELSPETH: The following morning, Dr. Ripley's brother, William, who was an assistant surgeon at a London hospital, having heard of the accident, came straightaway to see him.

[William stands.]

WILLIAM: James. You don't look so well. How's your leg?

DR. RIPLEY: It's been better.

WILLIAM: Where's your doctor? I'd like to speak to him.

DR. RIPLEY: Her.

WILLIAM: I beg your pardon?

DR. RIPLEY: Her. My doctor is a her, Dr. Verrinder Smith.

WILLIAM: What? You're pestered with one of *those*?

DR. RIPLEY: I don't know what I'd have done without her.

WILLIAM: No doubt she's an excellent nurse.

DR. RIPLEY: She knows her work as well as you or I.

WILLIAM: Speak for yourself, James. Besides, you know the principle of the thing is all wrong.

DR. RIPLEY: You think there's nothing to be said on the other side?

WILLIAM: Good heavens, no! Do you?

DR. RIPLEY: I don't know. It struck me during the night, we may have been a little narrow in our views.

WILLIAM: Nonsense, James. It's well and good for a woman to win prizes in the lecture room, but you know as well as I do they're no use in an emergency. I warrant this woman was all nerves when she set your leg. In fact, I had better just take a look at it and see that it's all right.

DR. RIPLEY: I'd rather you didn't undo it. I have her assurance that it's fine.

WILLIAM: Of course, if a woman's assurance is of more value than the opinion of the assistant surgeon of a London hospital, there is nothing more to be said.

DR. RIPLEY: I'd prefer you didn't touch it.

WILLIAM: Well, I shall see you soon, then. Good day, James.

[William sits.]

ELSPETH: *[To audience]* And he left. Doctor's brother is a fine surgeon, no doubt, but for all that, *[speaks in mock confidential tone to audience]* he's a bit of an ass. *[In mock innocence]* Oh, my, excuse me, that slipped out.

    Well, over the course of the next two months, Dr. Smith visited Dr. Ripley daily, and as time passed their visits grew longer. It became clear to me that Dr. Ripley found his personal physician rather interesting, though their conversations touched on many subjects I was hard pressed to follow. Of course, I just caught bits and snatches as I passed by his room, but it seemed that they found many areas of mutual interest, and discussed them on remarkably even terms. And not all of their conversations were on lofty matters . . .

DR. RIPLEY: I don't know how to apologize to you.

DR. SMITH: What about?

DR. RIPLEY: This woman question. I used to think a woman must lose some of her charm if she took up such studies.

DR. SMITH: Oh? You don't think they're necessarily unsexed, then?

DR. RIPLEY: Please don't recall my idiotic expression.

DR. SMITH: I am pleased I have helped in changing your views. I think that is the most sincere compliment I have ever been paid.

DR. RIPLEY: Well, it's the truth.

ELSPETH: And it certainly seemed to be. As it seemed to be true also that Dr. Ripley had become more than a little attached to Dr. Smith. As his convalescence progressed, her visits became more and more infrequent. And as the time between her visits increased, Dr. Ripley's mood swings, between elation at her presence and depression at her absence, became more pronounced. As the occasion for her final visit grew near, he seemed more and more sure that that visit was critical. When I showed her to his room, I saw an expression on his face I had never seen before. I excused myself, and on the way out noticed that the keyhole was in *desperate* need of polishing.

DR. RIPLEY: Verrinder, what a pleasant surprise. Do come sit by me.

DR. SMITH: Of course. You seem in high spirits today.

DR. RIPLEY: I am. For I have made a decision. I have decided to ask you to do me the honor of becoming my wife.

DR. SMITH: What, and unite the practices?

DR. RIPLEY: *[Hurt]* Surely you don't attribute such a base motive to me! I love you as unselfishly as ever a woman was loved!

DR. SMITH: I'm sorry. That was unkind of me. Forget I ever said it. Oh, James, I am sorry to cause you any disappointment, and I truly appreciate the honor you do me, but what you ask is quite impossible.

DR. RIPLEY: But . . .

DR. SMITH: I am so sorry. If I had known what you were thinking, I'd have told you earlier that I intend to devote my life entirely to science. There are many women with a capacity for marriage, but few with a taste for biology. I must remain true to myself. I came here, James, to wait for an opening in the Paris Physiological Laboratory. I have just heard there is a vacancy for me there, and so you will be troubled by my intrusion on your practice no more.

DR. RIPLEY: Verrinder . . .

DR. SMITH: No, James. I have done you an injustice just as you did me one. I thought you narrow and pedantic with no good quality, but I've learned during your illness to appreciate you better, and the recollection of our friendship will always be a pleasant one to me. Farewell, James.

ELSPETH: *[To audience]* And she left. In less than two weeks. *[Pause]* And once again there is but one doctor in Hoyland. One doctor who looks a good deal older than he did before, who seems a bit sadder than he ever did before, and who is less concerned than ever with the eligible young ladies that chance, or careful country mothers, place in his way. Good evening.

END

QUESTIONS FOR DISCUSSION

This story was written in the 1890s at a time when more and more women were becoming physicians in the United States and in England. Doyle quite accurately reflects the views of many male physicians who recoiled at the idea of female physi-

cians. Articles written at the time used the very same arguments — physiological as well as social — that the Ripley brothers do in this story to keep women out of the profession. Many women took the tack of the fictional Verrinder Smith, choosing career over family. Others opted to marry, have families, and practice medicine. Nowadays half or more of medical students in the United States are women.

Some of the issues that this story raises also arise in Susan Mates's "Laundry."

Were you surprised at the ending? Did you like the ending? How would you change it? Why?

What does Verrinder Smith mean by: "I must remain true to myself"?

Do women sacrifice more than men to become physicians (or to have any career)? What dilemmas do women physicians face in their careers and families when they try to do both?

Do you sense a bias against women in medicine? In other professions?

What is the significance of the differing reactions to Verrinder Smith of Thomas, William Ripley (James's brother), and the townspeople?

How many people in the audience have female physicians?

Do you think the entry of large numbers of women into the profession has altered medicine?

Do you think that there are some medical specialties that are better suited to women than others?

Has medicine "masculinized" women who become physicians, as some of the characters in the story suggest?

Is Dr. Ripley a "wimp"? Why didn't he just try harder to compete with Dr. Smith, by, for instance, doing surgery?

Why did Dr. Ripley change his mind about women physicians? Or did he?

Is it really possible that Verrinder Smith was surprised by James's declaration of love? How could she miss the signs of it?

Is this story outdated and quaint? Or does it have relevance to today's world?

PART IV. AGING AND CHRONIC ILLNESS

◎ ◎ ◎ ◎ ◎

He

KATHERINE ANNE PORTER

Adapted for Readers' Theater by Gregory A. Watkins

CAST
Mr. Whipple (Mr.)
Mrs. Whipple (Mrs.)
Doctor (Dr.)
He

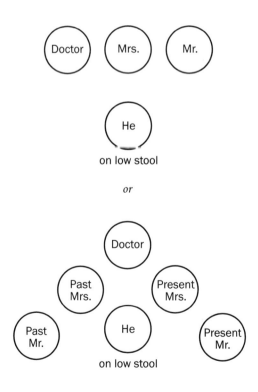

NOTES

Either in the program or during the introductions, the audience should be informed that (1) the story takes place in early summer on a small Southern farm during the 1920s; (2) the action shifts freely between the present (early summer) and the past, and the readers (except He who remains seated throughout the story) will indicate a shift to the past by standing when flashbacks take place; (3) the words He says aloud in the performance are actually He's thoughts, because He is unable to speak; and (4) He is in another room, separate from the adults (who are in the kitchen [He calls it "the food room"]), on a low cot.

If desired, the cast may include a Mr. and Mrs. Whipple from the past and a Mr. and Mrs. Whipple from the present. The former two characters speak the lines in the sections indicated by the words "[shift to the past]."

When characters stand to indicate a flashback, they should position themselves at a 45-degree angle from their seats. Their eyes should focus offstage in the direction in which they are standing.

He sits by himself on a low stool or crate throughout the performance. He talks like a young child though he is older than that, and may make appropriate childish movements as he speaks his lines.

If a male is not available to play He, a female can read this role. (We have done it and it works fine!)

HE: *[In pain]* Hot. Real hot. And my legs hurt. Bad. Mama's in the food room. I wish she would make me feel better.

MR.: Doctor's here.

MRS.: Already? He weren't supposed to be here so early.

MR.: Well, he's here.

MRS.: Is Mr. Taylor with him?

MR.: Don't see 'im.

MRS.: Well, how are we supposed to get to the hospital? Doctor said Mr. Taylor was gonna bring his carryall to take us to the hospital.

MR.: Reckon he'll be along presently.

MRS.: Well. I certainly hope so.

MR.: Morning, Doc. C'mon in.

DR.: Morning, folks. How are you?

MRS.: Where's Mr. Taylor?

DR.: He'll be along. Cow got sick and he had to fetch the vet.

MRS.: Well, I hope he gets here soon. I'm like to change my mind.

MR.: Now, Ma.

MRS.: You hush!

DR.: I understand how you feel, Mrs. Whipple. I got a boy of my own. But you'd better listen to me. I can't do anything more for him, and that's God's own truth.

MRS.: But . . .

DR.: *[Interrupting]* It's better you put Him in the County Home, for treatment, and right now. He'll have good care and be off your hands.

MRS.: We don't begrudge Him any care. And I will not let Him out of my sight. I won't have it said I sent my sick child off among strangers.

DR.: I know how you feel.

MRS.: It's just charity. That's what we've come to, Pa — *charity*. I won't have it. Lord knows I never looked for it.

MR.: We pay taxes to help support the place, just like everybody else, and I don't call that taking charity. I think it'll be fine having Him where He'll get the best of everything. And besides, I can't keep up with these doctor bills any longer.

MRS.: Maybe that's why the Doctor wants us to send Him — he's scared he won't get his money.

DR.: Now, Mrs. Whipple.

MR.: Hush, woman.

MRS.: *[Pause]* All right. But He won't stay long. Soon as He's better again we'll bring Him home.

DR.: Mrs. Whipple, I've told you time and again He can't ever get better.

MRS.: *[With fire]* Doctors don't know everything!

HE: Mama, I'm hot. My legs hurt. Please, Mama.

DR.: *[Brightly]* Well, how're your other young'uns? Adna and Emly?

MR.: *[Joining in]* Adna's working over to Powell's Grocery Store. And Emly's working at a railroad eating house over in Millersville.

MRS.: *[Almost detoured]* I think Emly's gonna come home for a vacation this summer, and Adna can get down for weekends. We'll all work together and get on our feet again, and the children will feel they've got a place to come home to.

DR.: Good, good. Uh, did Emly finish school?

MRS.: She'll finish soon. For now her wages are good, and she gets her food, too. The way the farm's been, that's a blessing.

MR.: *[Tired of this]* The farm's fine.

MRS.: No it ain't. It gets worse every year.

MR.: *Woman!*

MRS.: It does.

MR.: Hush!

MRS.: You're always getting cheated. Three years ago, you traded off one of our plough horses for a new one and a little money, so's we could buy groceries, and the new horse died of the heaves. Lord, but that was a hard winter.

MR.: Weren't that hard.

HE: Hot. So hot. Bees in my ears.

DR.: Was that when He first took sick?

MRS.: It was cold. Bitter cold. Adna and Emly had a four-mile walk to school, and Pa said:

[All shift to past — Mr. and Mrs. stand.]

MR.: Let 'em have *His* overclothes. He sets around the fire a lot. He won't need so much.

MRS.: *[Unsure]* That's so, I guess. And when He does outside chores he can wear your tarpaulin coat. I can't do no better.

HE: *[Confused]* Cold. Chest hurts. Hard to breathe.

[Dr. stands.]

DR.: Howdy, folks

MRS.: Look at Him, Doctor, He's almost blue. We've done everything we know how, but He just don't get no better.

DR.: Well, keep Him warm and give Him plenty of milk and eggs. He ain't as stout as He looks, I'm afraid. You got to watch 'em when they're like that. And put more cover on Him.

MRS.: *[Lying]* I just took off His big blanket to wash. I can't stand dirt.

DR.: *[Knows it]* Well, you put it back on the minute it dries. He'll get pneumonia.

MRS.: Get the blanket off our bed, Pa, and put His cot in by the fire. They can't say we didn't do everything for Him, even to sleeping cold ourselves on His account.

[Shift back to present — all sit.]

DR.: When that winter broke, He seemed to be well again, though I remember His feet seemed to hurt Him a bit.

MR.: He run the cotton planter that season.

DR.: I swear, 'til that boy took sick I durn near come to believe He was indestructible.

MR.: Remember when that plank blew off the chicken house and fetched Him upside the head?

MRS.: I almost died of fright. And He weren't even hurt.

MR.: Don't believe He even knew He'd been hit.

MRS.: And the way he used to skitter around in the trees. Like a regular monkey.

[He shifts to past — remains seated.]

HE: So high! I'm up so high. Like a bird. A big, white, pretty bird.

MR.: Could climb higher'n Adna. And Him so fat. Great rolls of fat, like an overcoat.

MRS.: Hush, Pa. No, He never got hurt, never got sick. Emly was forever getting bruised, and Adna couldn't fall a foot without cracking a bone, but He could do anything and not get a scratch. Preacher said such a nice thing once when he was here. He said, and I'll remember to my dying day, "The innocent walk with God — that's why He don't get hurt."

HE: So high. Like a bird.

MR.: Strong, too. He could carry twice as much wood and water as Adna.

DR.: Really? Well, you were lucky with His health. Emly always had colds, I remember.

MRS.: Head colds. She takes that after me. Take one in a minute. So in bad weather we'd give her the extra blanket off His cot. He never seemed to mind the cold. *[Realizes what she's said.]* Oh Lord.

DR.: *[Quickly]* It's not your fault He got sick, Mrs. Whipple. He was a strong, healthy boy. You had no reason to believe He'd ever be otherwise.

MRS.: The neighbors warned me. They warned me I needed to watch over Him better.

MR.: *[Bitterly]* Heard one to say, "It'd be a mercy if He should die. It's the sins of fathers."

MRS.: *[Angered]* They was always watching everything He did, talking like I weren't taking care of Him right.

[Mr., Mrs., and He shift to past — Mr. and Mrs. stand.]

MRS.: Oh, I do mortally wish they would keep out of our business. I can't afford to let Him do anything for fear they'll come nosing around about it. Look at the bees, now.

HE: Pretty. Pretty to see, pretty to hear.

MRS.: Adna can't handle them, they sting him up so. I don't have time to do everything, and now I don't dare let Him, for fear they'll see it. *[Pause]* If He gets a sting, He don't really seem to mind.

MR.: He ain't got sense enough to be scared of anything.

MRS.: You ought to be ashamed of yourself, talking that way about your own child. Who's to take up for Him if we don't, I'd like to know?

MR.: All I meant was . . .

MRS.: He sees a lot that goes on. He listens to things all the time.

HE: Pretty to see, pretty to hear. Like Mama.

MRS.: And anything I tell him to do, He does it. Don't never let anybody hear you say such things about Him. They'll think you favor the other children over Him.

MR.: At least I don't favor Him over them.

MRS.: What?

MR.: You're always telling folks you love Him so much. More'n your other two put together. More'n your whole family. You make people think nobody has feelings about Him but you.

MRS.: It's natural for a mother. You know it's more natural for a mother to be that way. People don't expect so much of fathers, somehow.

MR.: How 'bout what Adna and Emly expect?

[Shift back to present — all sit.]

HE: Hot. So hot. Bees all in my ears.

DR.: Where is He now?

MR.: Asleep in the other room.

MRS.: He was running a fever again, so we laid Him down and covered Him.

HE: Oh, hot.

DR.: Has He had anything to eat? It's a long ride to the County Home.

MR.: Wouldn't eat nothing this morning.

MRS.: I tried to get Him to take some biscuit and egg, but He wouldn't have none of it. It hurts so to see Him like this. He used to love to eat.

[He shifts to past — remains seated.]

HE: Goodgoodgoodgooodgooooodgoooooooood.

MR.: Wouldn't cry for food like the others. Just took what you give Him, went and squatted in the corner and ate, smacking His lips and mumbling.

HE: *[Singsong]* This is nice, this is nice, I like happy, this is nice.

[He shifts back to present.]

MRS.: He'd eat all of His and whatever the rest of us left. 'Course, that weren't often much. Not around here.

MR.: We had plenty left that night we wasted a pig on your brother and his family, didn't we?

MRS.: You can be so mean-spirited. I don't get to see my family but once in a blue moon, and I just wanted to show them we were doing fine.

MR.: At the cost of three hundred pounds of pork, when we hardly had enough to feed our own.

MRS.: All you did was complain. Wouldn't even help butcher the pig, you nor Adna neither.

[Mr. and Mrs. and He shift to past — Mr. and Mrs. stand.]

MR.: All right, do it yourself, then. Christamighty, no wonder we can't get ahead.

MRS.: And how am I supposed to get that little pig away from his Ma? She's a fighter, worse'n a Jersey cow. *[Calls out.]* Adna?

MR.: No use there. Boy's afraid of the old sow.

MRS.: All right, then. *[Pause]* Watch *Him* do it. He's not afraid. *[To He]* Bring me that little pig, would you, Honey. You'll do that, won't you? Mama wants it for a special treat. Go on now.

HE: C'mere little pig, pretty pig. C'mere. Mama wants you for a special treat. C'mere little pig.

MR.: Run, boy. That old sow's charging you.

HE: Uh oh, uh oh, big pig's mad. Runrunrunrunrunrunrun.

MRS.: Thank God, thank God. Oh, I'm so proud of you, Honey. Now, hand him here and step back. Don't want to get no blood on you.

HE: Blood?

MRS.: Gimme your knife, Pa. I want a good, clean cut.

HE: Cut?

MRS.: There.

HE: NO! Nonononononono. Little pig. Runrunrun.

MRS.: What's the matter, Honey?

HE: Gotta go away. Go now. My stomach hurts. So bad.

MR.: *[Pause]* Don't worry, Ma. He'll forget. And eat plenty, just the same.

MRS.: *[Disturbed]* He'd eat it all if I didn't stop Him. He'd eat up every mouthful from the other two, if I'd let Him.

[Shift back to present — all sit.]

MRS.: Next morning I dropped everything to get Him all cleaned up. In an hour He was dirty again, with crawling under fences after a possum.

[He shifts to past — remains seated.]

HE: C'mere possumpossumpossum. Oh fun. Pahhhh-sssummmmmmm.

MRS.: That, and straddling along the rafters of the barn, looking for eggs in the hayloft.

HE: *[Singsong]* This is nice, this is nice, I like eggs, yum yum yum.

MRS.: I told Him to get out of His dirty clothes, and I . . . I boxed both His ears. Hard.

HE: *[Surprised]* Mama?

MRS.: He didn't cry — He didn't make a sound — but the look on his face . . .

HE: *[Hurt]* Mama?

[He shifts back to the present.]

MR.: He forgot about it, Ma. He forgets everything. But He wouldn't come eat with her brother's family, no sir. Can't say as I shouldn't have joined Him.

MRS.: *[Subdued]* We all had a very nice visit. And He didn't eat with us, but he ate. I took Him a heaping plate before anyone else got *any*.

MR.: *[Sarcastic]* A very nice visit.

MRS.: *[Rising to the bait]* Everybody had plenty to eat. And my brother and his family were so polite. No out-of-the-way remarks. I get awfully sick of people's remarks.

MR.: It's easy to be polite when you come to eat. Who knows what they had in their minds?

MRS.: That's just like you.

DR.: I wonder what's keeping Mr. Taylor.

HE: Hot, hot, hot.

MRS.: I hope he never comes.

MR.: Now, Ma.

MRS.: It ain't right. He's our child.

HE: I don't feel good, Mama.

DR.: Mrs. Whipple, He's sick. And He's not going to get any better — ever. But the folks at the County Home can take care of Him. He'll have a good chance to be comfortable and happy.

MRS.: *[Searching]* But how'll we run the farm without Him?

DR.: Mrs. Whipple, He's been bedridden for four months now, since He had that fit. He can't be any help around here the way He is, and He's not going to get any better.

MRS.: I don't know.

MR.: He's right.

HE: Mama, please make me feel better.

DR.: And even if I never charged you anything, He'll be needing medicine all the time from now on, medicine the County Home can provide for Him.

MR.: *[Pause]* He's sick, Ma. You've done all you can. If you try to do anymore, *you'll* get sick.

MRS.: No.

MR.: Remember the bull? The one Jim Ferguson lent us to breed our cow late last summer?

MRS.: I was so embarrassed. You shouldn't have let him know we were as down as that.

MR.: We had to send *Him* to fetch the bull because I needed Adna to help me in the field.

[Mrs. and He shift to past. Mr. remains in the present. Mrs. stands.]

MRS.: That's a good idea. Adna's too jumpy. You got to be steady around animals.

MR.: It was a hot day, and a three-mile walk, but He took even longer than you thought he should have.

MRS.: It's just like everything else in life. I'll never know a moment's peace about anything.

MR.: You called me in from the field. Worried sick.

MRS.: He should be back by now.

MR.: Then we saw Him turn into the side lane, limping along real slow.

MRS.: He's hurt.

HE: I'm tired. Hot. The sky is pretty.

MR.: He was leading the bull by a ring through his nose, twirling a little stick in His hand.

HE: *[Singsong]* This is nice, this is nice, I won't drop it, this is nice.

MR.: He never looked back, or sideways, just walked along with his eyes half shut, twirling his stick.

MRS.: I've heard about bulls. They'll follow on quiet enough, and then pitch on with a bellow and paw and gore a body to pieces.

MR.: You froze right where you stood.

HE: I can make the stick go real fast.

MRS.: Any second now that black monster's gonna come down, and He ain't got sense enough to run.

MR.: Just then, the old bull heaved his head and horned the air at a fly.

MRS.: RUN! RUN! For God's sake . . . please.

HE: I can make it go the other way too. Funfunfun.

MR.: You bolted right straight into the house.

MRS.: Lord, don't let anything happen to Him, please. You know people will say we oughtn't to have sent Him. You know they'll say we didn't take care of Him. Keep Him safe, Lord. Please. And I'll look after Him better, I swear. Amen.

HE: I could do a bigger stick, too. I'm strong.

MR.: The bull followed the boy, gentle as a lamb, right into the barn. I found you in the kitchen, in your rocking chair, with your apron over your head, rocking and sobbing away.

[Shift back to present — Mrs. sits.]

MRS.: I can't take it anymore.

MR.: You've done all a soul can do. But He needs help now. And the County Home can give it to Him.

MRS.: No more.

DR.: Mr. Taylor's here. *[Long pause]* Mrs. Whipple?

MRS.: I'll fetch Him.

DR.: Are you sure? *[Long pause] [To Mr.]* Is she all right?

MR.: I reckon. She'll have to be.

MRS.: *[To He — Mrs. walks over to He.]* Hello, Honey.

HE: Mama? Please make me better.

MRS.: I've got a surprise for you, Honey. We're gonna go for a ride in Mr. Taylor's carryall. Isn't that nice?

HE: So hot. Bees in my head.

MRS.: Did you hear me, Honey? We're going for a ride.

HE: Don't wanna ride. Wanna stay here. Wanna feel good.

MRS.: We're going to a real nice place. You'll like it.

HE: This is nice, this is nice. I will stay here, this is nice.

MRS.: Come along now, Honey. Let's go for a ride.

HE: Don't wanna ride. Want my mama. Mama?

MRS.: Come along now. Honey? What are you doing? Oh, dear God. Are you crying?

HE: Mama?

MRS.: You're not crying, are you, Honey? Lord, you never cried about any-thing in your whole life. Please don't.

HE: Mama?

MRS.: You don't feel so bad, do you, Honey? Please stop. You're not thinking about the bull, are you? Or about sleeping cold and not being able
to tell me? Or about that time I boxed your ears? Please, God, make
Him stop.

HE: I want my mama.

MRS.: Look, Honey. It's just gonna be for a little while. 'Til you're better.
Then you can come home and we will all be happy again. Please.

HE: Gotta find my mama. Let's go. Gogogogogogogo.

MRS.: There's a good boy. Come along now. *[Mrs. walks back to seat.]* And
please stop crying.

HE: Gotta find Mama. This is nice, this is nice, find my mama, this is nice.

END

QUESTIONS FOR DISCUSSION

How does Mrs. Whipple feel about He? How does she show how she feels?
How does she deal with her feelings? Does she love He more than the
rest of the family, as her husband suggests?

Why is Mrs. Whipple so reluctant to send He to the County Home?

What is the turning point of the story? Does Mrs. Whipple change in the
story?

Is Mrs. Whipple a sympathetic character?

Why doesn't He have a real name?

Is He aware of what is going on around him? What does the evidence
indicate?

What do you make of the story's ending? Why is it so dramatic? Why
is Mrs. Whipple so surprised when He starts to cry at the end of the
story?

What is this story about?

What is the physician's role in the story? Mr. Whipple's role? Are these two
characters unfeeling toward He and the situation the Whipples are in?

Is Mrs. Whipple a good mother?

Did the Whipples do the right thing by sending He to the County Home?

How is this story relevant to today? What issues does this story raise about
  care of the chronically ill? What impact does chronic illness have on
  family dynamics? Does chronic illness strengthen or weaken family
  relationships?

Why is He always capitalized in the story?

If the Whipples had more money, would the story be different? Is class an
  issue in the story?

A Mistaken Charity

MARY E. WILKINS FREEMAN

Adapted for Readers' Theater by Gregory A. Watkins

CAST

Magistrate
Miz Simonds
Charlotte
Harriet
Widow Mills
Sheriff
Nurse Allen
Mr. Simonds
Miz Thomas
Mr. Hood

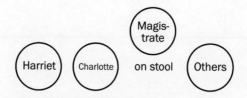

NOTES

This story may be performed and discussed along with the shorter "Management." There are a lot of small roles in this script. Using different voices and positions (i.e., standing for one character and sitting for another), one person can play two (or even more) roles. Possible pairings of roles include: Magistrate and Mr. Hood,

Miz Simonds *and* Miz Thomas, Widow Mills *and* Nurse Allen, Sheriff *and* Mr. Simonds.

Charlotte *pronounces* Harriet's *name with the accent on the last syllable. Both* Charlotte *and* Harriet *could be portrayed with "country" accents.*

This story, though poignant, is also humorous and will draw some laughter from the audience at certain points in the script.

Magistrate *sits on a stool, higher than the other readers who sit in regular chairs. When addressing* Magistrate, *the characters face angled stage left about 45 degrees. When they interact with* Charlotte *and* Harriet, *they face angled stage right about 45 degrees. They always maintain offstage eye focus.* Harriet *and* Charlotte *always face straight forward toward the center of the audience and maintain offstage eye focus.*

MAGISTRATE: All right, let's get started. Now, first, I want to make it clear we're not here to fix blame, nor to find fault. We just need to clarify what happened, and decide what we're going to do next. Miz Simonds, I believe you're most familiar with the Shattucks, and this situation. Perhaps you could get us started.

MIZ SIMONDS: *[Stands, addressing Magistrate]* Thank you sir. When all this began, Harriet and Charlotte, the Shattucks, were living west of town, in their little, low, weather-stained cottage at the end of an old dirt footpath. They had themselves a bit of land, mostly gone to seed, and a little garden. They're both terribly old and, as you know, Harriet's almost deaf, and Charlotte's blind. They worked a very meager, very difficult livin' out of the land.

CHARLOTTE: Is there enough for a mess, Harriét? *[Pause. Then louder, because her sister is hard of hearing.]* Is there enough for a mess, do ye s'pose, Harriét?

MIZ SIMONDS: I don't know how many times I went out to pay a call on 'em, to find Harriet on her hands and knees in the garden, pullin' dandelion greens. To eat.

HARRIET: Well, I don't know, Charlotte. There's plenty of 'em here, but I ain't got near enough for a mess; they do boil down so when you get 'em in a pot; an' it's all I can do to bend my joints enough to dig 'em.

CHARLOTTE: I'd give consider'ble to help ye, Harriét.

MIZ SIMONDS: Charlotte was almost always on the doorstep, in an old chair. The doorstep is sunk low down in the grass, and the whole house looks to be settling down and moldering into the grass as into its own grave. When Harriet grew deaf and rheumatic, and had to give up her work as a tailoress, and Charlotte lost her eyesight and was unable to do any more sewing, Mr. Morgan, who holds a mortgage on their house, gave them the use of it, rent and interest free. He might as well have taken credit to himself for not charging a squirrel for his tenement in some old decaying tree. Honestly, it's hardly a house anymore. Rain and snow filter through the roof, mosses grow over it, worms eat it, and birds build their nests under its eaves.

WIDOW MILLS: *[Stands, addressing Magistrate]* Your honor?

MAGISTRATE: Yes, Miz Mills?

WIDOW MILLS: The Shattucks have always been poor people and common people; no especial grace and refinement or fine ambition has ever characterized any of them; they have always been poor and coarse and common. The father and his father before him lived in the poor little house, grubbed for their living, and then died. Their mother was of no rarer stamp, and the two daughters are cast in the same mold.

MIZ SIMONDS: After their parents died, Harriet and Charlotte lived alone in the old place.

MAGISTRATE: Neither of them ever married?

WIDOW MILLS: No.

SHERIFF: *[Clears his throat]*

MAGISTRATE: Sheriff.

SHERIFF: *[Stands, addressing Magistrate]* Not to be indelicate, but Harriet has a reputation for bein' a bit, well, blunt. Almost surly. And Charlotte always had the reputation of not being any too strong in her mind.

MIZ SIMONDS: Harriet used to go house to house doing tailorwork, and Charlotte did plain sewing and mending for the neighbors. They made enough to get by, but after Charlotte's eyes failed her, and Harriet had the rheumatic fever, and their savings went to the doctors, times were harder with them.

SHERIFF: They kept a roof over their heads, and food on the table, and it didn't seem like they suffered much.

MAGISTRATE: Yes, well. How did they get along once they couldn't work?

MIZ SIMONDS: When they couldn't pay the interest on the mortgage, they were allowed to keep the place interest free. Their neighbors, mostly farmers, and good friendly folk, helped them out with their living. One would donate a barrel of apples from the harvest, one a barrel of potatoes, another a load of wood for the winter fuel, and many of the farmers' wives took 'em a pound of butter, or a dozen fresh eggs, or a nice bit of pork. And there's the garden patch behind the house, with a struggling row of currant bushes, and one of gooseberries, where Harriet manages to raise a few pumpkins, which are the pride of her life. On the right of her garden are two old apple trees, a Baldwin and a Porter, both still in a tolerably good fruit-bearing state.

SHERIFF: Harriet's right proud of her pumpkins. The apples and currants, too. It's their own.

WIDOW MILLS: Miz Simonds carried them food, too.

[Sheriff and Widow Mills freeze. Miz Simonds addresses sisters.]

MIZ SIMONDS: *[Loudly]* Good morning, Harriet. I've been frying some doughnuts, and I brought you over some warm.

CHARLOTTE: I've been tellin' her it was real good in her.

HARRIET: Good mornin', Miz Simonds. *[Critical — doesn't want to show weakness]* Doughnuts, eh? *[Pause]* Tough. I s'posed so. If there is anything I 'spise on this earth it's a tough doughnut.

CHARLOTTE: *[Embarrassed]* Oh, Harriét!

HARRIET: They are tough. And if there is anything I 'spise on this earth it's a tough doughnut.

MIZ SIMONDS: *[Laughing]* Well, Harriet, I'm sorry they're tough, but perhaps you'd better take them out on a plate, and give me my basket. You may be able to eat two or three of them if they are tough.

HARRIET: They are tough — turrible tough.

MIZ SIMONDS: I suppose your roof leaked as bad as ever in that heavy rain day before yesterday?

HARRIET: It was turrible. Turrible. We had to set pails an' pans everywheres, an' move the bed out.

MIZ SIMONDS: Mr. Upton ought to fix it.

HARRIET: There ain't any fix to it; the old ruff ain't fit to nail new shingles on to; the hammerin' would bring the whole thing down on our heads.

MIZ SIMONDS: Well, I don't know as it can be fixed, it's so old. I suppose the wind comes in bad around the windows and doors, too?

HARRIET: It's like livin' with a piece of paper, or mebbe a sieve, 'twixt you an' the wind an' the rain.

MIZ SIMONDS: You ought to have a more comfortable home in your old age.

HARRIET: [Alarmed] Oh, it's well enough. The old house'll last as long as Charlotte an' me do. The rain ain't so bad, nuther is the wind; there's room enough for us in the dry places, an' out of the way of the doors an' windows. It's enough sight better than goin' on the town.

MIZ SIMONDS: Oh, I didn't think of your doing that. We all know how you feel about that, Harriet, and not one of us neighbors will see you and Charlotte go to the poorhouse while we've got a crust of bread to share with you.

HARRIET: [Relieved] Thank ye, Miz Simonds. I'm much obleeged to you an' the neighbors. I think mebbe we'll be able to eat some of them doughnuts even if they are tough.

MIZ SIMONDS: Good. Bye, now. [Turns back toward stage left, still standing, and freezes]

HARRIET: Bye.

CHARLOTTE: [Troubled] My, Harriét, what did you tell her them doughnuts was tough fur?

HARRIET: Charlotte, do you want everybody to look down on us, an' think we ain't no account at all, just like beggars, cause they bring us in vittles?

CHARLOTTE: No, Harriét.

HARRIET: Do you want to go to the poorhouse?

CHARLOTTE: *[Frightened]* No, Harriét.

HARRIET: Then don't hinder me agin when I tell folks their doughnuts is tough an' their pertaters is poor. If I don't keep up an' show some spirit, I sha'n't think nuthin' of myself, an' other folks won't nuther, and fust thing we know they'll kerry us to the poorhouse. You'd 'a been there before now if it hadn't been for me, Charlotte.

CHARLOTTE: *[Pause]* Did you get a good mess of greens, Harriét?

HARRIET: Tolerable.

CHARLOTTE: They'll be proper relishin' with that piece of pork Miz Mann brought in yesterday. O Lord, Harriét, it's a chink!

HARRIET: Humph.

CHARLOTTE: *[Hurt]* I guess that if you was in the dark, as I am, Harriét, you wouldn't make fun an' turn up your nose at chinks. If you had seen the light streamin' in all of a sudden through some little hole that you hadn't known of before when you set down on the doorstep this mornin', and the wind with the smell of the apple in it came in your face, an' when Miz Simonds brought them hot doughnuts, an' when I thought of pork an' greens jest now — O Lord, how it did shine in! An' it does now. If you was me, Harriét, you would know there was chinks.

HARRIET: Why, Charlotte, hev it that thar is chinks if you want to. Who cares?

CHARLOTTE: Thar *is* chinks, Harriét.

HARRIET: Well, thar's chinks, then. If I don't hurry, I sha'n't get these greens in in time for dinner.

MIZ SIMONDS: *[To Magistrate]* That was when I knew what we had to do. It's not fit for anyone to have to live like that, especially in their old age.

WIDOW MILLS: Miz Simonds came to me, and we discussed how we might help the poor Shattuck women. We decided it would be best to help them move to a place where they could be looked after, where they could have proper food, shelter, and clothing. Fortunately, there was an opening at the Old Ladies' Home.

MAGISTRATE: Nurse Allen, that's your establishment, isn't it?

NURSE ALLEN: *[Stands, addressing Magistrate]* Yes, sir. Miz Simonds and

Widow Mills came to us at a fortuitous time. We had had a very difficult spring, with an unusually high mortality. There were a number of
vacancies, and we were delighted to welcome the Shattucks.

MIZ SIMONDS: Widow Mills was gracious enough to pay the entrance fees,
and Nurse Allen made the arrangements quickly and comfortably.

NURSE ALLEN: *[Nods and sits]*

MAGISTRATE: So the Shattucks moved into the Home.

MIZ SIMONDS: Well, they were a little reluctant.

SHERIFF: A little? I believe you had to call on the Reverend to help convince
them.

MIZ SIMONDS: Yes, they were a *bit* reluctant. Understandably. They'd lived
in that old house of theirs all their lives, and I'm sure they were a bit
concerned about the change. But once we shared with them all the
benefits of the move, they agreed.

WIDOW MILLS: Harriet was particularly swayed when Miz Simonds
pointed out how much more comfortable Charlotte would be with the
extra care. Charlotte's blind, after all.

MIZ SIMONDS: Their biggest fear seemed to be that the Home was some
sort of almshouse. Once we convinced them that that wasn't the case,
they agreed.

SHERIFF: But they still weren't especially happy to go.

MAGISTRATE: Mr. Simonds, you helped them move, didn't you?

[Mr. Simonds stands, addressing Magistrate. Widow Mills and Sheriff sit.]

MR. SIMONDS: Yes, sir.

MAGISTRATE: How did they take it?

MR. SIMONDS: Neither was very happy. Charlotte cried for a while, right
pitiful. It was a sad sight to see, those two little old ladies in their wore-
out dresses, with their poor old clothes box.

MIZ SIMONDS: *[Disagreeing]* They were fine.

MR. SIMONDS: I took them to the depot. The missus was there, and the
widow, and Nurse Allen. Everybody seemed real happy about things,
except the Shattucks.

MIZ SIMONDS: They were nervous.

MAGISTRATE: Undoubtedly.

MR. SIMONDS: When I saw 'em all there, together, I couldn't help rememberin' a passage from Scriptures, about how it's "more blessed to give than to receive."

MAGISTRATE: Yes, of course. Nurse Allen, the Shattucks were comfortable at the Home?

[Nurse Allen stands; Mr. Simonds sits.]

NURSE ALLEN: Yes, sir. Oh, there was a period of adjustment, but that's fairly common amongst new arrivals. We serve a fine cuisine at the Home, particularly our soups, and they may have found that a bit strange at first.

CHARLOTTE: O Lord, Harriét, when I set down to the table here there ain't no chinks. If we could have some cabbage, or some pork an' greens, how the light would stream in!

NURSE ALLEN: And we ask that all our residents dress cleanly and comfortably. Not that the Shattucks were untidy.

MIZ SIMONDS: Widow Mills generously provided Harriet and Charlotte with new black cashmere dresses, white lace caps, and lovely neckerchiefs. Both ladies seemed very pleased with their new wardrobes.

NURSE ALLEN: In fairness, they did seem a bit uncomfortable in the new clothing. Almost as if they felt they were violating the Sabbath by wearing them on weekdays.

MAGISTRATE: Miz Thomas, you spent as much time with the Shattucks as anyone. Did they seem comfortable in their new surroundings?

[Miz Thomas stands, addressing Magistrate. Miz Simonds and Nurse sit.]

MIZ THOMAS: Comfortable enough, your honor, but, to be honest, I'm not sure anything could have transformed the Shattucks into two nice little old ladies. They did not take kindly to the lace caps and neckerchiefs. They told me they felt as if they broke a commandment when they put them on every afternoon. They had always worn calico with long aprons at home, and they wanted to still. They wanted to put their hair up and go without caps, just as they always had done. Charlotte in a dainty white cap was pitiful, but Harriet was both pitiful and comical. They just didn't seem to fit in, and they felt it, as people of their stamp always do. No amount of kindness and attention—and they had enough of both—seemed to help.

CHARLOTTE: O Lord, Harriét . . .

MIZ THOMAS: And Charlotte blasphemed so, though she didn't seem to know it.

[Miz Thomas sits.]

CHARLOTTE: Let's go home. I can't stay here no ways in this world. I don't like their vittles, an' I don't like to wear a cap; I want to go home and do different. The currants will be ripe, Harriét. O Lord, thar was almost a chink, thinking about 'em; an' the Porter apples will be gittin' ripe, an' we could have some apple pie. This here ain't good; I want merlasses fur sweeting. Can't we get back no ways, Harriét? It ain't far, an' we could walk, an' they don't lock us in, nor nothin'. I don't want to die here; it ain't so straight up to heaven from here. O Lord, I've felt as if I was slantendicular from heaven ever since I've been here, an' it's been so awful dark. I ain't had any chinks. I want to go home, Harriét.

HARRIET: *[Pause as she decides on a plan of action]* We'll go tomorrow mornin', then. We'll pack up our things an' go; we'll put on our old dresses, an' we'll do up the new ones in bundles, an' we'll jest shy out the back way tomorrow mornin'; an' we'll go. I kin find the way, an' I reckon we kin git thar even if it is fourteen mile. Mebbe somebody will give us a lift.

[Sheriff and Nurse Allen stand.]

SHERIFF: And that's apparently what they did.

NURSE ALLEN: We found their caps, one on each post at the head of the bedstead.

SHERIFF: Near as I can tell, they took their bundles, snuck out, and took off down the road, hobbling along, holding each other's hands, as happy as two young'uns. They were seen by several people, though no one took much notice of 'em.

[Nurse Allen sits.]

CHARLOTTE: *[Laughing]* O Lord, Harriét, what do ye s'pose they'll say to them caps?

HARRIET: *[Laughing]* I guess they'll see as folks ain't goin' to be made to wear caps agin their will in a free country.

MAGISTRATE: Sheriff? Two elderly women, one of 'em blind, just walked out of the city? Just walked away?

SHERIFF: Well, sir, the Home is right on the outskirts of town. A short walk brought them into free country road — though even here, at ten o'clock in the morning, there was considerable traveling to and from the city on business or pleasure. I talked to some of the folks who saw 'em walk out of town, and they said that, though they was worried at first at the sight of the two old ladies, Harriet, I guess, was moving along with such a sense of what she was about that they just shrugged it off.

MAGISTRATE: And they walked all the way home?

SHERIFF: No sir. Mr. Hood here was coming out of town in his wagon, and he saw 'em walking down the road.

MR. HOOD: *[Stands, addressing Magistrate]* I passed 'em real slow-like, and then pulled my team to a stop. They was quite a sight, the two of 'em.

SHERIFF: Mr. Hood did 'em a real good turn.

MR. HOOD: *[Turns stage right, addressing Harriet and Charlotte]* Like a ride, ma'am?

HARRIET: Thankee. We'd be much obleeged.

SHERIFF: He fetched 'em up in the wagon, an' set off down the road.

MR. HOOD: Seems to me you look pretty feeble to be walking far. Where were you going?

HARRIET: *[Defiantly]* Out to the Shattuck home.

MR. HOOD: *[Surprised]* That's fourteen miles out. You could never walk it in the world. Well, I'm going within three miles of there, and I can go on a little farther as well as not. But I don't see — have you been in the city?

HARRIET: I been visitin' my married darter in the city.

CHARLOTTE: *[This next exchange between the sisters should be in stage whispers.]* Harriét?

HARRIET: Charlotte?

CHARLOTTE: You ain't never told a deliberate falsehood in your whole life.

HARRIET: Charlotte, this here's one of them times that justify a little white lie, seems to me.

CHARLOTTE: But . . .

HARRIET: Seems to me we got no choice. If we ain't keerful, this young feller jest might turn directly around and carry us right back to the Home. You want to go back to them caps?

MR. HOOD: I shouldn't have thought your daughter would've let you start for such a walk as this. Is this lady your sister? She's blind, ain't she? She don't look fit to walk a mile.

HARRIET: *[Defiantly]* Yes, she's my sister, an' she's blind, an' my darter didn't want us to walk. She felt real bad about it. But she couldn't help it. She's poor, an' her husband's dead, an' she's got four leetle children.

SHERIFF: *[Laughing]* She told Mr. Hood one heck of a story, all without battin' an eye. Seems her poor daughter had had one pitiful time of it.

MR. HOOD: Well, I'm glad I overtook you, for I don't think you would ever have reached home alive.

NURSE ALLEN: Oh my goodness! We passed them! On our way out to their house. Once we discovered that they'd gone, an attendant and I took a coach and rode out to their house. We passed an old wagon on the way. I didn't even see them.

HARRIET: *[Stage whisper]* Squinch down, Charlotte.

CHARLOTTE: *[Stage whisper]* What?

HARRIET: *[Stage whisper]* It's that lady from the Home. Squinch down.

MR. HOOD: *[Turns, addressing Magistrate again]* Yeah, I seen a wagon go past us. Anyway, I let 'em out at the head of the path to their house, an' watched as they walked up it.

SHERIFF: That's how they got home.

[All sit.]

MAGISTRATE: Remarkable.

HARRIET: The clover is up to our knees. An' the sorrel and the white-weed; an' there's lots of yaller butterflies.

CHARLOTTE: O Lord, Harriét, there's a chink, an' I do believe I saw one of them yaller butterflies go past it!

HARRIET: Come on in the house. I'll see if I can't find us somethin' to eat.

CHARLOTTE: O, Harriét.

HARRIET: An' don't git to weepin'. We're home. *[Pause]* Goodness, the currants are ripe, an' them pumpkins have run all over everything.

CHARLOTTE: O Lord, Harriét, thar is so many chinks that they're all runnin' together!

END

QUESTIONS FOR DISCUSSION

Is "A Mistaken Charity" an apt title for this story? Why? Was this a mistaken charity? Do you think Miz Simonds, Widow Mills, and the other neighbors are overly paternalistic toward the Shattuck sisters or just doing what was right and necessary? Could the sisters' situation have been handled another way?

What are the "chinks" Charlotte sees at home but not in the Home? What do the chinks mean?

Why is Harriet so tough-sounding toward those who try to help her and her sister?

Why were Harriet and Charlotte unhappy in the Old Ladies' Home?

What should the magistrate decide in this case? What should be the next step for the sisters, the neighbors, the community?

Is there a class issue embedded in this story? What bearing might class have on the way the sisters were treated? Do class issues influence our care of the elderly?

What should be the role of physicians, of families, of society, in situations like this?

What experiences from your own life does this story bring to mind?

Is this a sad story or a happy one?

Do you think the story would have been different if the two protagonists had been men instead of women?

Management

MARGARET LAMB

Adapted for Readers' Theater by Gregory A. Watkins

CAST

Mail Carrier

Bitsy Larkin (Bitsy)

Bank Teller (Teller)

Welfare Investigator (Welfare)

Robber

Mrs. Frazer (Frazer)

James Taylor (Taylor)

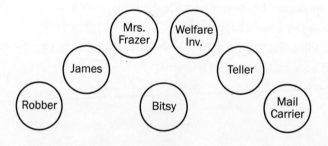

NOTES

This story is short and may be performed and discussed along with "A Mistaken Charity." Bitsy and Miz Frazer are African American in the original story. Mr. Taylor's and Welfare Investigator's race or ethnicity are not stated. Robber could dress in all black.

MAIL CARRIER: On the first of the month everyone is out on the stoop early, looking for *me*. I carry the mail. All along the block people stand or sit, talking or just waiting. Most of them are on welfare; some of them never get any mail except their half-monthly check. It's certainly the only mail Bitsy Larkin ever gets.

BITSY: I been on the city roll since it began. I didn't have work, nobody had work, and they give out food tickets and clothes, not money.

MAIL CARRIER: No one knows how old she is, not even Bitsy. I asked her once and she said . . .

BITSY: Weren't never told. But I was born in freedom.

MAIL CARRIER: Even on a sunny day, wearing two or three sweaters, Bitsy still shivers with cold. She's so old and thin she's always cold. One of her eyes is so blind it's blue, and the other one is getting cloudy. Still, she's active. As soon as I give her the check she shoves it in her pocket and takes off for the bank. Same thing every check day.

TELLER: She comes into this bank twice a month. Walks the three blocks from her house. She stands in line, patiently, until she reaches my window. Then she takes out her check and a pen, and signs her name *very* carefully, as if she's copying from a picture she has in her head. Then she fishes around in her pockets to find her identification card.

BITSY: How much, Miss?

TELLER: Fifty-one dollars and fifty-five cents.

BITSY: Thank you.

TELLER: She always seems relieved, as if she's afraid one day the check will be for less.

WELFARE: We in the Welfare office keep tabs on her expenses. Twenty-six dollars for her room at Miz Frazer's, one-half month's rent. The rest is for the food she cooks in Miz Frazer's kitchen, a few clothes she puts in Miz Frazer's laundry bag (for which she pays extra), and whatever else she might need before the next check.

BITSY: I always go straight home from the bank, to put aside my rent money. I don't want to be put out. Some people can't live on their welfare cause they eat the rent, then the landlord wants his money and they get put out. 'Sides, I don't eat so much nowadays. And I'm careful with my money. I get along.

ROBBER: She always comes straight home from the bank. It was easy. Everybody else is out spending their checks, and the old woman is there by herself. And I didn't really hurt her. I just pulled her hands out of her pockets and she dropped the money right on the floor. She fell down by herself. If she hadn't tried to get up, I wouldn't even have had to kick her.

BITSY: My side! It feels like when I broke my hip. Oh, Jesus. Help me, please.

ROBBER: Somebody will help her, when they get back.

BITSY: After a while I could stand up. I unlocked Miz Frazer's door and went into her kitchen, but she wasn't there.

FRAZER: I was in New Jersey, to visit my sister.

BITSY: I was real hungry, but I just couldn't eat Miz Frazer's food. And I had already ate all my food the night before, to make room for new groceries. I buy 'em every check day.

FRAZER: I found her the next day, when I got back from New Jersey. She was laying on her mattress, crying. She'd been there since the day before. When she told me what happened I told her to get right down to the Welfare office and get another check. She can't live without money.

WELFARE: She seemed terrified when she came into my office. It must have been a tough experience for her. In fact, I don't think I'd have been able to understand what had happened to her without the notes from the doctor and the police.

BITSY: They wanted to keep me in the emergency room, but I told them I had to see the Welfare.

WELFARE: I asked her if Miz Frazer would wait for the rent.

BITSY: *[Pause]* Hard to say.

WELFARE: So I called Miz Frazer myself, and explained the situation to her.

FRAZER: No, I wouldn't put her out — if y'all give me your word on the rent. I need it this week. I'm a widow, and that's my income. I'll tell you what else, too. Miz Larkin is a very peculiar person. I don't know if I should keep on with her, a person of her age. Too much responsibility for me.

WELFARE: I told Miz Larkin we would cut her another check, and got her some food money for three days. Two dollars and ninety-five cents. I asked her if she could get home all right.

BITSY: I'm growing foolish, child, but I ain't a baby yet.

TELLER: I was surprised to see Miz Larkin at the bank again so soon, but not as surprised as she was by the fact that the check was for a different amount than usual.

WELFARE: The cash we issued had to be deducted from the check.

BITSY: They know what they're doing. But I still ran out of food two days before the next check. Guess my appetite was up.

FRAZER: She pretended to be sick, like she couldn't eat. I told her I was gonna call a doctor, but she said . . .

BITSY: No. I'll be on my feet tomorrow.

MAIL CARRIER: I brought her her regular check on the sixteenth, and she set straight out for the bank.

BITSY: I cashed my check, bought me some chicken parts to cook, and went straight home.

ROBBER: Like clockwork. It was easy. This time she didn't even try to resist. Smart lady.

BITSY: Lord, I just want to die.

FRAZER: Robbed again. I took her right down to that Welfare office and I told *them* to look after her. I have my own troubles, scuffling hard, looking for rent. I can't carry her over here every time.

WELFARE: Now, Miz Larkin, don't cry. Let's try to think what's best. Do you have any relatives? *[Pause]* Did you ever have any children? *[Pause]* Were you ever married? *[Pause]* Miz Larkin, our records are confused. First you say you have children, then you say no kin at all.

BITSY: That's a different time. It don't matter no more. I got to concentrate on what I'm doing *now*. To live.

WELFARE: You don't have anyone?

FRAZER: I don't see no need for questions. Bitsy don't even know her Christian name. Why don't y'all take and put her in a nursing home where she belongs. If a person can't help themselves, that's where you send them. She'd get the best help there.

BITSY: No. Please.

WELFARE: Miz Larkin seems to have a management problem. We'll work it out.

FRAZER: I don't want her in my house no more.

WELFARE: We want Miz Larkin where she will be happiest. *[Pause]* I had Miz Larkin and Miz Frazer wait while I cut another check. Then I gave the check to Miz Frazer. She was to deduct the rent, then give Miz Larkin her food money daily.

FRAZER: I didn't like it. I don't want nothing to do with welfare money. I reminded Miz Larkin that the welfare people ain't forgotten about the nursing home.

BITSY: A nursing home is like the hospital. When I broke my hip, they took away my clothes and things so I couldn't see them, and I had to lay in a big room with lots of beds and people always crying.

TAYLOR: I was helping Miz Larkin's super load a washing machine into a wheelbarrow when I heard her neighbors talking about what had happened to her. After a while they all went in to supper, and Miz Larkin came out on the stoop. I went up and introduced myself:

Good evening, Miz Larkin. I'm James Taylor.

BITSY: Good evening.

TAYLOR: Sorry to hear about your troubles.

BITSY: Uh-huh.

TAYLOR: Miz Larkin, this house just ain't no good for you, with the junkies waitin' on your check. I was thinkin' I might be some help to you.

BITSY: They're gonna put me in a nursing home.

TAYLOR: Well, a friend of mine has a nice room empty. No junkies there. Maybe you could go see it.

BITSY: I don't know. It's getting dark.

TAYLOR: Come on. It's only a few blocks away, and I'll walk you back after. It's a nice room. *[Pause]* And you won't have to go to no nursing home.

BITSY: *[Reluctantly]* Okay.

TAYLOR: I suppose Miz Frazer charges fifteen dollars a week for that little bitty room.

BITSY: Uh-uh.

TAYLOR: More? Less?

BITSY: She takes twenty-six dollars out of my every check.

TAYLOR: And makes you climb all those stairs? The room you're gonna see is on the first floor.

BITSY: [Pause] The house don't look so bad. Old, but not so bad. [Pause] And the room seems kind of empty. Just a cot, a chair, and a little table.

FRAZER: At my house she had a big bed with a headboard, a big old chair with lots of pillows, and a chest with a mirror.

BITSY: Mr. Taylor, it don't have no window. Miz Frazer got a window looks right down on the street.

TAYLOR: You see how clean it is here. No dirty people here.

BITSY: [Pause] It is clean.

TAYLOR: And here you don't have to worry about Miz Frazer or no nursing home.

BITSY: Well . . .

TAYLOR: I'll tell Mr. Andrews you'll move in on the first. You just explain to the Welfare you'll be living with a family. That way they don't have to fill out no papers. And don't tell Miz Frazer you're moving until we have the money safe in hand.

BITSY: I ain't sure about the bathroom in the hall. And the kitchen is upstairs. That's not the way it is at Miz Frazer's.

TAYLOR: They'll be fine. You'll be fine. You just have to listen and learn how to get along with the Welfare. They won't send you to no nursing home.

MAIL CARRIER: [Pause] On the first, Miz Larkin and Mr. Taylor met me several blocks from Miz Frazer's, back along my route, and asked for her check.

BITSY: I want to get to the bank early.

MAIL CARRIER: I didn't like Mr. Taylor too much, but it's her check, so I gave it to her. They took off back along my route, I guess to avoid Miz Frazer's.

BITSY: This ain't my bank.

TAYLOR: It's okay. Just give the man your check.

BITSY: Fifty-one dollars and twenty-six cents? That ain't right.

TAYLOR: This man gets paid a quarter to cash your check. Look, you don't want to do the way you done the last two checks — went to the bank and got your money stole. Here, let me hold it for you.

BITSY: I don't feel so good. Kinda cold and sick.

TAYLOR: Now, you tell the Welfare you took your whole check and moved this mornin' to a new room. That's the truth, too. Here's the address: "Andrews family," so they knows you the *sole* lodger. Tell them you already moved and paid out twenty dollars for the truck. That way they be sure to give you the money. I needs the money before so's I can get ahold of that truck. The movin' company name is right here on this card, with the telephone. Then you ask for new dishes, pots and pans, since you ain't going to use Miz Frazer's no more. The Andrews family uses all they own. You understand?

BITSY: Pots and pans?

TAYLOR: The new rent is fifteen dollars a week. So now you paid a week's rent, a week's security, and the movin' expenses. That's fifty dollars. Here's the receipts all wrote out to show them.

BITSY: I need food money.

TAYLOR: They're gonna give it to you, honey. You got legitimate expenses. Now go on over to the Welfare while I start to work on the moving. I got to get home in case the Welfare calls. And remember, you're gonna move away from the people who take your money. You won't need no nursing home. You'll be safe.

WELFARE: She brought me the receipts, and told me about Mr. Taylor and her move. I was a little worried that the rent was higher . . .

BITSY: I'll be safer.

WELFARE: And that Mr. Taylor was so eager to get his money . . .

BITSY: He's the only one to help me.

WELFARE: But everything seemed to be in order. I wanted to go with Miz Larkin, to look at the new room, but I had two other emergencies to deal with and she seemed to have things under control. I talked the situation over with my supervisor and we decided to cut Miz Larkin the checks — and cancel the nursing home memo. I did warn her that if she had any more problems she'd *have* to go to the nursing home.

FRAZER: Then she shows up at my house with no rent.

BITSY: Ain't no rent. Fixin' to move out.

FRAZER: And she went to her room and packed. I asked her where she was moving but she wouldn't say. Just kept right on packing. I made sure she just took her own things — two old lamps, an old coat way too big for her, some quilts, an old radio, a pile of shoes, and her church certificate. I asked when she was leaving.

BITSY: Mr. Taylor gonna pick me up before supper.

FRAZER: Then you owe me rent since noon. *[Pause]* And Mr. Taylor didn't show up 'til after eight. Pulling some nasty old fruit cart.

TAYLOR: Couldn't get a truck, but this'll do fine for your little bit.

FRAZER: I guess they ain't never too old, Mr. Taylor. Maybe I'll call up the Welfare —

TAYLOR: After the way you treated this lady —

FRAZER: But it ain't none of my business. I'm quit of her. *[Pause]* He loaded her things in the cart and they took off down the street.

BITSY: I sure hope things'll be better now.

TAYLOR: *[Disinterested]* Uh-huh.

BITSY: Welfare gave me the checks, just like you said.

TAYLOR: You let me hold them for you.

BITSY: *[Giggles]* They safe now. They hid good. And I ain't undressin' in the street.

TAYLOR: This old coat comes from the garbage. You ask the Welfare, they give you a new one.

BITSY: The Welfare don't want to give too much.

TAYLOR: They give you the checks today.

BITSY: The Welfare only let me stay by myself if I ain't gonna bother them too much. That's what they said. They tole me if my money gets stolen again I got to go to the nursing home. They tole me "Miz Larkin, anytime you get unhappy you come right on over." They got that bed ready for me. I tole them I ain't decided yet — maybe yes, maybe no. I just needs my few bitty things. Once I goes into that nursing home the checks stop for good. Nothin' for nobody.

TAYLOR: I could find you a bargain on those pots and pans.

BITSY: You can help *some*. A person don't need but so many pots and pans.

TAYLOR: You're gonna do fine, Miz Bitsy.

END

QUESTIONS FOR DISCUSSION

This story is based (partially) on an incident in the author's life when she was a social investigator at the Harlem Welfare Center. Discussion questions below include some that can be used for comparing and contrasting the events, characters, and issues in "Management" and "A Mistaken Charity."

The story is called "Management." Whose management problem is it?

Is there a medical problem here? Who is responsible for aging people without families like Bitsy? Is this a government responsibility? A community responsibility?

Does Bitsy belong in a nursing home? Who should decide where she belongs? Is the system managing Bitsy well?

Is Miz Frazer being too hard by wanting Bitsy out? Does she want Bitsy out?

Is Mr. Taylor a bad guy? Who is he? What does he want? Why is he helping Bitsy? Does he help her?

What do you make of the ending of the story?

Is Bitsy managing? Is she getting taken? Is she getting the support of the community? Of society?

Is race an issue in the story? In the original story, Miz Frazer is African American, as is Bitsy. Neither Mr. Taylor's nor the welfare investigator's race is stated (though the author told the editor of this readers' theater anthology that the former is meant to be African American and the latter is meant to be white). Would you interpret the story any differently if Miz Frazer were white or Mr. Taylor or the welfare investigator were one race/ethnicity or another?

How would you compare and contrast the community support of Bitsy in "Management" and of the two sisters in "A Mistaken Charity"?

An underlying theme in both stories is the matter of retaining dignity and self-worth in times of vulnerability. Do the aging protagonists in these two stories succeed in this regard? How?

What appears to be the future of Bitsy? Of the two sisters? If you see a difference in outlooks, why?

What issues regarding care of the aged in our population do these stories raise?

How do factors like race, gender, culture, community, and economic status affect the elderly in these two stories and in American society?

Biographical Notes

PEARL S. BUCK (1892–1973), the Nobel Prize–winning writer, is known for her stories and novels about Asia.

SIR ARTHUR CONAN DOYLE (1859–1930), best known for his Sherlock Holmes stories, was also a well-trained physician who practiced medicine for a number of years before turning to full-time writing.

MARY E. WILKINS FREEMAN (1852–1930) wrote many stories and a few novels, primarily about women and mostly set in New England, her home region.

MARGARET LAMB (b. 1936), who teaches English at Fordham University, has written short stories, novels (including *Chains of Gold*), plays (including *Monkey Music*), and a history of Shakespeare on stage (*"Antony and Cleopatra" on the English Stage*).

SUSAN ONTHANK MATES (b. 1950) retired from clinical medicine and teaching in Providence, Rhode Island, in 1997 to devote herself full-time to writing and other interests.

KATHERINE ANNE PORTER (1890–1980), who is probably best known for her 1962 novel *Ship of Fools*, often wrote stories about life in the South. In 1966 she won the Pulitzer Prize and the National Book Award for her *Collected Stories*.

RICHARD SELZER (b. 1928) is a retired surgeon and full-time writer of stories and essays primarily about medicine who for many years practiced in New Haven, Connecticut, where he still lives.

WILLIAM CARLOS WILLIAMS (1883–1963), physician and world-renowned poet who practiced medicine for fifty years among the working-class citizens of Rutherford, New Jersey, wrote a number of short stories that used his experience in medicine to explore the lives of physicians and their patients.

Permissions

tor Stories (New York: Picador USA). Adapted for readers' theater with permission of Georges Borchardt, Inc., for the author.

Readers' theater adaptation of "The Girl with a Pimply Face" is based on a story by William Carlos Williams from *The Collected Stories of William Carlos Williams*, copyright 1938 by William Carlos Williams. Used by permission of New Directions.

"He" was first published in 1927 and appeared in Katherine Anne Porter's 1930 collection of short stories, *Flowering Judas* (New York: Harcourt, Brace). Permission to adapt and perform the story as readers' theater was granted by Barbara Thompson Davis, Literary Trustee for the Estate of Katherine Anne Porter, c/o The Permissions Company, High Bridge, N.J.

"Imelda," copyright © 1982 by David Goldman and Janet Selzer, Trustees, appeared in Richard Selzer, *Letters to a Young Doctor* (New York: Simon & Schuster, 1982), and was reprinted in his 1998 short story collection, *The Doctor Stories* (New York: Picador USA). Adapted for reader's theater with permission of Georges Borchardt, Inc., for the author.

"Laundry" was published in Susan Mates's 1994 collection of short stories, *The Good Doctor* (Iowa City: University of Iowa Press). Adapted for readers' theater with permission of the author and the University of Iowa Press.

"Management" by Margaret Lamb was first published in the feminist literary magazine *Aphra* (1971) and reprinted in *Solo: Women on Woman Alone* (New York: Delacorte Press, 1977), edited by Linda Hamalian and Leo Hamalian. Adapted for readers' theater with permission of the author.

"A Mistaken Charity," originally published in Mary E. Wilkins Freeman, *A Humble Romance and Other Stories* (New York: Harper & Bros., 1887), has been reprinted in numerous anthologies, including *The Revolt of Mother and Other Stories* (Old Westbury, N.Y.: Feminist Press, 1974), edited by Michele Clark. The story is in the public domain.

Readers' theater adaptation of "Old Doc Rivers" is based on a story by William Carlos Williams from *The Collected Stories of William Carlos Williams*, copyright 1938 by William Carlos Williams. Used by permission of New Directions.

Readers' theater adaptation of "The Use of Force" is based on a story by William Carlos Williams from *The Collected Stories of William Carlos Williams*, copyright 1938 by William Carlos Williams. Used by permission of New Directions.